SUDOKU PUZZLE BOOK

OVER 500 PUZZLES FOR ADULTS & KIDS INCLUDING: EASY, MEDIUM, HARD, EXPERT & EXTREME

SUDOKU DELUXE BOOKS CREATION & INSTRUCTION TEAM

Table of Contents

Sudoku Explanation

Sudoku is a logic based, numerical placement puzzle. It is played on a 9x9 grid with the numbers 1-9. The object is to fill the grid so that each row, column, and 3x3 subgrid contains each of the numbers 1-9.

Each puzzle will start with some of the numbers filled in, such that the puzzle only has one solution. As the puzzles go up in difficulty there will be less and less numbers supplied to start with. Let's look at an example of an easy puzzle below.

	3			9				1
		2	3		5			9
6	9	7	2			4		5
		4	9				8	
	5		7			2		3
7	8	3	5		1			4
			1					8
5	4		6	7				
2		1					4	6

This puzzle already has 36 of its 81 numbers filled. This includes several columns that are only missing 2 numbers. These can be a nice place to start. Let's look at the far right most column first. It is missing a 2 and a 7. The puzzle below shows the spaces that we are going to fill in first as well as one more space that is important.

	3			9				1
		2	3		5			9
6	9	7	2			4		5
		4	9				8	
	5		7			2		3
7	8	3	5		1			4
			1					8
5	4		6	7				
2		1					4	6

We know that the far right column is missing a 2 and a 7. We also know that due to the rules of Sudoku, that the 7 cannot be in the bottom space because a 7 already appears in that row. So, we can fill in the puzzle as follows.

	3			9				1
		2	3		5			9
6	9	7	2			4		5
		4	9				8	7
	5		7			2		3
7	8	3	5		1			4
			1					8
5	4		6	7				2
2		1					4	6

We can continue to use logic like this until we fill in the entire puzzle. Just remember that each puzzle has only one possible solution, but there may be many ways to arrive at that solution. Try to find what works best for you and go with that.

Best of luck and happy puzzling!

EASY

Puzzle #1 - Easy

4	7	2	3	8	6	9	1	5
9	3	1	2	5	7	6	4	8
5	8	6	4	9	1	2	3	7
7	4	5	9	3	8	1	6	2
3	2	9	6	1	5	8	7	4
1	6	8	7	2	4	3	5	9
8	1	7	5	6	9	4	2	3
6	5	3	8	4	2	7	9	1
2	9	4	1	7	3	5	8	6

Puzzle #2 - Easy

7	4	5	8	3	2	6	9	1
3	2	9	4	6	1	5	7	8
6	1	8	7	9	5	3	4	2
2	8	6	3	7	4	9	1	5
1	7	3	2	5	9	8	6	4
6	5	4	1	8	6	7	2	3
8	9	1	6	4	3	2	5	7
4	6	7	5	2	8	1	3	9
5	3	2	9	1	7	4	8	6

Puzzle #3 - Easy

2	3	8	7	1	9	6	5	4
7	6	4	5	3	8	2	9	1
1	5	9	4	2	6	3	8	7
3	9	2	6	8	4	7	1	5
6	4	1	2	7	5	9	3	8
5	8	7	1	9	3	4	2	6
4	2	6	3	5	1	8	7	9
8	7	5	9	6	2	1	4	3
9	1	3	8	4	7	5	6	2

Puzzle #4 - Easy

2	4	9	3	1	6	7	5	8
1	8	3	4	7	5	2	9	6
6	7	5	2	9	8	3	1	4
8	5	4	9	2	3	1	6	7
9	6	7	5	8	1	4	3	2
3	1	2	6	4	7	9	8	5
5	9	8	7	3	4	6	2	1
7	3	1	8	6	2	5	4	9
4	2	6	1	5	9	8	7	3

Puzzle #5 - Easy

1	7	3	9	8	2	5	6	4
4	6	9	3	7	5	8	2	1
2	8	5	4	6	1	3	7	9
8	3	6	2	4	7	9	1	5
7	2	4	5	1	9	6	3	8
9	5	1	6	3	8	2	4	7
6	9	2	7	5	4	1	8	3
5	1	7	8	2	3	4	9	6
3	4	8	1	9	6	7	5	2

Puzzle #6 - Easy

9	6	2	1	3	4	5	7	8
4	1	8	9	7	5	2	3	6
3	7	5	6	2	8	9	1	4
7	5	1	3	8	9	4	6	2
2	3	9	4	6	7	8	5	1
8	4	6	5	1	2	3	9	7
1	8	4	7	5	3	6	2	9
6	2	3	8	9	1	7	4	5
5	9	7	2	4	6	1	8	3

Puzzle #7 - Easy

4	9	7		3	2			8
8	6							
			8	1			6	
9	7	3	1			6	8	
6	2							
				7			2	4
					1	8		
1		9		8	3	7	4	
	8	2		6	9	5	1	

Puzzle #8 - Easy

		3		4		9		
1	6		3	9			4	2
					7			
5	3		8				6	1
	9	4		5		2		7
7		8	6	2		3	9	
					5			
	5	7	4	8		6		3
4			7				5	

Puzzle #9 - Easy

					5			1
	1			3	7	4		
4		2	9				5	3
2	7		5		4			
			7	2		9	8	
1		9				2		5
9				6	3		2	
	3	7	8			1		9
		1		7				

Puzzle #10 - Easy

	4	2		9			8	7
9	7					6		4
8	5		7					
			9		1	5	6	
		6		5	7		4	3
1			4		2			
		9	5		8			
4	6			2				
						9	3	8

Puzzle #11 - Easy

6	1			8	2	9		
	9							
	5	2		4	9	6		
		3		5	8	2	7	
		8		2	3		9	4
							3	
	8				4		1	2
4	3			9			6	
2		5		1	7	3		9

Puzzle #12 - Easy

	8	2	4		1			6
		4					8	
	6		7	8	5			
		7	8		6		3	1
	1							8
			3	1	9		2	
2	7				8	6	9	
	3		9		2		7	
6	9		1			8	4	

Puzzle #13 - Easy

				4			8	
4	1		8	2		6		
7	5	8	6					
3	9	1					2	
			1			8		
8	6			7		1	3	
1			9		6		4	8
	8		7		2		9	6
9	2		3				7	

Puzzle #14 - Easy

5		1		9	6	8		2
7		4		3	8		1	9
8				1				
	8			2	3	9	4	7
						6	8	
		6	8		1			
						2	6	
	4	2			7			
6		8	1			7	9	3

Puzzle #15 - Easy

3					1			8
7		1	9				5	
		8	7			9		6
		7	4	9				1
	1	9			7			5
	4		6				9	
	5				6	8	4	
4	8		3					7
1				4	2		6	

Puzzle #16 - Easy

4							9	
2		6		1		7		
	3		7		9		4	6
1	4			3	7			
	8	5				1		4
			8		1	9	7	
6		4			5			9
	7		6	8		5	1	
		8	9					

Puzzle #17 - Easy

8		3	4		7		2	9
5		2		9	1		8	4
		4	2		9			
7	3	9	1	6				
2					3		9	6
			8	3		9	1	5
3		8			5			2
				4	2		6	

Puzzle #18 - Easy

	1		3	7			4	
2		3				7		
6	7	5		2				1
	5	2	6					
4	8	7		3				6
9					7	8		3
				6	3		9	8
1		8					6	7
	9	6		4	1			

Puzzle #19 - Easy

				2	6			
		4			3	1		9
1		3	9				6	5
6	8	9	2		7		5	
4	5		6	3	8	2		
2			3	7		5		4
	4			6			3	1
	9	8						

Puzzle #20 - Easy

		7	1			9		4
	1	9	5				7	
	4				9			6
		8	6	9				7
7		1			5			9
3			8				1	
1					6	4	2	
4	8		7					3
	5			8	4		6	

Puzzle #21 - Easy

		7	8		4			3
	4		7	5			1	
		5		3	9		6	
		8	2		5		9	4
5						7		
	7	4	6	8			3	
		3		1	7		2	
		6	3		2			9
	5		9	6			4	

Puzzle #22 - Easy

8				7		6	9	
1		7		9				5
		3			1	8		
	4			6				9
9	1				7	5		
7			9	4		1		
	8	4		3		7		
		1	4		2			6
	5				6		8	4

Puzzle #23 - Easy

3	9	1						2
8	6		7				1	3
					1		8	
4	1		2		8		6	
7	5	8			6			
			4					8
1				6	9	8		4
9	2				3			7
	8			2	7	6		9

Puzzle #24- Easy

	1		8	9			4	
			5	7	4		6	
6					2	9		
		5		6				9
4		6			8			3
3				4	7			8
5					9		2	
	4	9	7			5		
7	2	1				8		

Puzzle #25 - Easy

1						9	2	8
9		2		3		7		5
		7	2					
		5	7	1		6		2
			5			3	7	4
7				6				
3			9			8		1
8	5		3		1			7
6	7		8		5	2		

Puzzle #26 - Easy

9					2		5	3
1			3			9		
5	4		9	6	7			2
3	2		5					7
4			8	7	3		1	5
		8			4			9
8								1
			4	5		7		6
6		4		2	1			

Puzzle #27 - Easy

							6	8
8			3	2		7	9	4
	6		1		8			
							2	6
4	2		7					
	8	6			1	3	7	9
	4	7	8	3		9		1
		8		1				
	1	5	6	9		2	8	

Puzzle #28 - Easy

				7			4	2
3	9	7			1	6		8
	6	2						
2		8	9	6		5		1
			1			8		
9	1		3	8		7		4
				1	8			6
7	4	9	2	3			8	
	8	6						

Puzzle #29 - Easy

		3	4				5	7
	8		5		7	9		
7		6			2			3
		9	2	1		4		
	3		7					1
1	7			9		2		
	9			5		3	1	
	1			2	9			4
		2			8	5		

Puzzle #30 - Easy

1				8	4	9	6	
		8		6	9	7	2	
9		2			7	3		
4		1	6			8		2
7	8	5				6		
					8			4
			8			1		
3	1	9			2			
8		6	1		3			7

Puzzle #31 - Easy

		3			9			1
7	6	9		2			4	5
2			5	3				9
3	7	8	1	5				4
		5		7			2	3
4				9		8		
1	2					4		6
	5	4		6	7			
				1				8

Puzzle #32 - Easy

2	5		6				7	
1			7		2	4	3	
	4		9	3			8	5
			4					2
6		8	5	1	9		4	3
4						8		
	6	1	2		3	9	5	7
	7			9				
					5		1	

Puzzle #33 - Easy

4		8	7				3	
1					6	4		2
		5		8	4			6
3			8					1
	8		6	9			7	
7	1				5		9	
		4			9		6	
	9	1	5					7
	7		1			9	4	

Puzzle #34 - Easy

	8	4		2	5	1	9	
	2	9		3	8	7		4
		2		8	3	5		
	6					2	4	
9	1	5					3	8
			3	9	7		6	1
	9	6			2	3		
				4		9		2

Puzzle #35 - Easy

6	2				7		1	
	4			9				
		3	6	4		9		7
				7	9	1		8
5		8	4		1			
	1	4				7	3	
8								9
4	6		9			5		
		7		1	5		8	6

Puzzle #36 - Easy

	2	7	3				5	8
		3						
4		9	8				2	3
				9				
	9			1	6		8	2
	6		2	5			4	9
		6		3	4		9	
2		1		8				4
9	3		5		2		1	7

Puzzle #37 - Easy

			1	3		7		
		3					6	
	2	7	4	6				3
7						8		
		4		9	6			
	1			8	7	3		6
	7	1	9				5	8
3	5		6		8		2	7
2	6				1	9		4

Puzzle #38 - Easy

		2	5			8	3	
9	1	5		8	3			
	6		2		4			
	2	9	7	4		3	8	
	8	4	1		9	2	5	
				1	6	9	7	3
			9	2		4		
	9	6	3				2	

Puzzle #39 - Easy

6	8			1	5		7	
		5	9			6		4
9								8
	1				7	2		6
7		9	6	4			3	
				9		4		
			4		1		8	5
8		1		7	9			
	3	7				1	4	

Puzzle #40 - Easy

8	7		6		3			
3			2			6	7	
6	2			9			3	
4	6			1			2	
5	8					4		9
	9			3	4			8
	5			6		3		
				5	9	1	4	
2					1		5	

Puzzle #41 - Easy

8			4	9			2	3
				3				
3				7	2		5	8
2	5				6		4	9
	1	6			9		8	2
	9							
	3	4		6			9	
5		2	9		3		1	7
	8		2	1				4

Puzzle #42 - Easy

	5	2	4	8		1		9
	8	3	9	2		7	4	
				6		2		4
	3	8	2			5		
			5	1	9		8	3
		4				9	2	
3	7	9					1	6
	2		6	9		3		

Puzzle #43 - Easy

						1	5	
3			1	6				
	2		7		5	3	8	9
5		8	2		4	7		1
7		9	6		3		2	8
		2			7			
9		1		7		8	6	3
						5	7	
2	7		5					

Puzzle #44 - Easy

	5		9				1	7
		8		1				3
9		6	7				8	
	6			2	4			1
8	4			6		5		
		7	3			8		4
	9		6			4		
		1	4		9		7	
		5		7		1	9	

Puzzle #45 - Easy

1		6	9			2	8	
5	2		6			9	4	
9								
3		4			6		9	
	5	2	3	9		7	1	
8				2	1	4		
					3			
	8			4	9	3	2	
	3		2		7	8	5	

Puzzle #46 - Easy

	9	4	8	5				
2			6	4			1	
	8		9				3	4
3			2	6			9	
7		6		3		2		
			7	8		6		3
5				2				1
4		1					5	9
		3	5				6	

Puzzle #47 - Easy

		8		1				
			7	6		4		5
	4	6					1	2
4		5		2		9	7	6
		9		3	5		2	
		1	9			3		
		4		5	1	8	3	7
	8			9			4	
2		3		7		5		

Puzzle #48 - Easy

		3		5	7			4
8			9			7		5
	7	6			3	2		
7	1		2				9	
		9	4				1	2
3					1			7
		2	5			8		
9			3	1			5	
1					4	9	2	

Puzzle #49 - Easy

	8	5	9				7	1
	7	2	6		8	3	5	
9	4				1	2	6	
8						7		
3	6			8	7		1	
				9	6			4
		6						3
	3		4	6			2	7
7			1	3				

Puzzle #50 - Easy

		1	6	9		8		4
	2	9		3				7
	8		2	7		6		9
8	5	7		6				
	1	4		8	2		6	
					4			8
				1			8	
1	9	3						2
	6	8			7		1	3

Puzzle #51 - Easy

1	9		5			7		
	7		1				4	9
4					9		6	
5				8	4	6		
8		4	7				3	
		1			6	2		4
	8		6	9			7	
	1	7			5		9	
		3	8			1		

Puzzle #52 - Easy

								9
	9			8	2	6		1
	6			4	9		2	5
9		4		2	3		8	
7	2			5	8		3	
3								
	3	9		1	7	2	5	
1		2			4			8
6				9		4		3

Puzzle #53 - Easy

		8		4				
	6		8	2		4		1
			6			7	8	5
8		4	9		6	1		
		7	3			9		2
6		9	7		2			8
	1	3		7		8		6
		2				3	1	9
	8		1					

Puzzle #54- Easy

3		4		6		9		
8			2	1			4	
	5	2	9		3	1	7	
5	2				6	4	9	
9								
1		6			9	8	2	
				3				
	8		4	9		2	3	
	3			7	2	5	8	

Puzzle #55 - Easy

6	9			4			5	
1		7		2				3
	3	2	9					6
					7	5		
	2	5	4	9				8
8	6			3			7	4
3		9		6				5
5	7			1			4	
	8	4	3					7

Puzzle #56 - Easy

		3	2				1	7
		6		9		3		2
	5		4			9	6	
5					7			
	7	4	3			6	8	
		8	9	4		2		5
		5	6				3	9
		7		3		8		4
	4		1			7	5	

Puzzle #57 - Easy

			8			2	1	7
		9		2				5
7			5			4	9	
8	9			4		1		
5	7	4		6				
		2	9					6
	6				9		5	
		8			3		6	4
	4	7			8			3

Puzzle #58 - Easy

3					5		6	
	5		2			1		
1	4					9	5	
4		9	5		8			
	2		4		6		1	
		8			9	4	3	
6	7		3					2
	3		6		2		9	
			8		7	3		6

Puzzle #59 - Easy

	7	8	6	3				
		3	2			6		7
	2	6			9			3
		2		1				5
				9	5	1		4
	5				6	3		
	9			4	3		8	
	6	4			1			2
	8	5				4	9	

Puzzle #60 - Easy

		4		9	8		1	
9			2			6		
		6	4	7	5			
8						7	2	1
		2	9			5		
5					7		4	9
	9			6				5
	8		7	4		3		
	3		8			4		6

Puzzle #61 - Easy

		3		9	6		2	
	2	9				4		
6	1					9	7	3
9		1		8	4	2	5	
	4	7		2	9	3	8	
		5			2	8	3	
4		2		6				
3	8		9	1	5			

Puzzle #62 - Easy

	2				4			
	3	4	1	9	5	8	6	
8							4	
		7			6		2	5
	5	8	3		9			4
4		3		2	7		1	
		1		5				
9	7	5		3	2	1		6
			9					7

Puzzle #63 - Easy

2	8		9	7		6	3	
			2				7	
	1	7	8	5		2	4	
				3		1		6
5		1						
8	9	3			2	7	5	
6	3	8	1	9				7
7		5						
				2	7	5		

Puzzle #64 - Easy

				3		6		
4	6		2	7			3	
1	3							7
6		8	5		3	2	7	
9			7	1		5	8	
		1	6		2		4	9
	8	7	1				6	3
	9	6		4				
					7			8

Puzzle #65 - Easy

8		7		3	9		2	6
	3	5	1		6			8
4	9		7	2			5	
		4			5			7
7	5		3	6			8	4
						5		
						7		
	6	1	2		4		9	3
3				9			4	

Puzzle #66 - Easy

1	9			7	3			8
		2	9			6	3	
				1		7		
	1						5	
	3	5	4	2				9
4					1	3	7	
2	5		1	9				
			2		7		4	5
9		8				2		7

Puzzle #67 - Easy

5	7		8	3	9		2	
			5	1				
	1	6						3
3	6		2		8	9		7
7						2		
4	2			7	1	8		5
		7	6	8	3	1		9
			7	5				
	5						7	2

Puzzle #68 - Easy

			9	8		2	7	
1	9		2		5			
2		7					5	4
9				2		6		3
	1					7		
	7	3	1		9		8	
		1	4			3		7
					1			5
4	2			5	3		9	

Puzzle #69 - Easy

	9		2				6	3
		1					7	
3		7		1	9	8		
7	2					5		4
	1	9		2	5			
			8	9		7	2	
1				4			3	7
	4	2	5		3	9		
					1			5

Puzzle #70 - Easy

6		3	9		7	2		8
		7	2					
2		4	8		5		7	1
	7		1		9	6	8	3
5				7	2			
						7	5	
7		5		2		8	3	9
1	6				3			
						5	1	

Puzzle #71 - Easy

2			6	3	8	4		5
		5	2		7	6	9	8
							8	9
5	4		3	7		2		
	1	3		6				4
				2	6			
	5	6	9			1	3	
1	9				3		4	

Puzzle #72 - Easy

		9		3	5		4	2
3	7		4			1		
	5			1				
			2	5			1	9
2		7	9		8			
	4	5				7	2	
		8	1	9		3		7
7								1
6	3				2		9	

Puzzle #73 - Easy

			3	9	7	6	1	
				4			2	9
6	9				2			3
	6					4		2
2				8	3			5
5	1	9				3	8	
9	2			3	8		4	7
4	8			2	5	9		1

Puzzle #74 - Easy

	7		3		1	8		5
		2	8		5	6		7
	1	8	9			3		
7	4	3	5					
				6		7		
	2	6	7	1			5	
2	8	9				1		
			2				7	
	5	7		3		9	2	

Puzzle #75 - Easy

5		4	3		7			2
	3	1			6	4		
						9	8	
				6	2			
	6	5	9				3	1
1		9		3			4	
	5		2	7		8	9	6
2			6	8	3	5		4

Puzzle #76 - Easy

	5		3					6
			1		4		9	5
		2			5		1	
	6	4			2			1
	9			8			4	3
	8	5	4	9				
	2	6			3			9
	7	8				6	3	
		3	6		7	2		

Puzzle #77 - Easy

		3						
4		9		8			3	2
	2	7		3			8	5
			9					
	9		1		6		2	8
	6		5	2			9	4
		6	3		4			9
2		1	8				4	
9	3			5	2		7	1

Puzzle #78 - Easy

9		1	5	2			8	4
	4	7	8	3			2	9
		5	3	8				2
3	8					9	1	5
4		2					6	
		3	2				9	6
	2	9		4				
6	1		7	9	3			

Puzzle #79 - Easy

	7						4	2
		1	3	9	7	6		8
				6	2			
1						8		
9	6		2		8	5		1
3	8		9	1		7		4
	1	8						6
				8	6			
2	3		7	4	9		8	

Puzzle #80 - Easy

2		4	9				8	7
	9	7				6		4
	8	5		7				
	1			4	2			
				9	1	5	6	
6			5		7		4	3
	4	6	2					
9				5	8			
						9	3	8

Puzzle #81 - Easy

		4		7	5	3		
2				3		6	7	
7		5	9					8
	5		3		1			9
9	2			4				1
8			5			2		
	1	2	4			9		
	9		2				1	7
		7		1				3

Puzzle #82 - Easy

1						8		
	7		6	8		1	3	
			9	3	1		2	
9		6		1			4	8
3			2	9			7	
7		2	8				9	6
	4						8	
8	2		1	4		6		
6			5	7	8			

Puzzle #83 - Easy

6		2	3				9	
8		7				3		6
3			7		6			2
2			5			1		
			4		1	9	5	
		5			3		6	
4		6	2				1	
		9		8		4	3	
5		8		9	4			

Puzzle #84 - Easy

				3		6		
	3	1					7	
	6	4		7	2			3
		9		1	7	5		8
8		6	3		5	2		7
1			2		6		9	4
7	8				1		3	6
			7				8	
6	9			4				

Puzzle #85 - Easy

		3	8	4	7			6
7				9		8		3
	6		5		2			
				2	3	7		
		2	7	6	5			1
	3	7	1				4	
				1	8		6	7
3		6					9	8
1		4	9		6			

Puzzle #86 - Easy

		2		8	3			5
1	9	5				3	8	
6						4		2
2		9		3	8		4	7
8		4		2	5	9		1
				4			2	9
9		6			2			3
			3	9	7	6	1	

Puzzle #87 - Easy

				9	6		4	
	3	6		8	7	1		
	8							7
2		7	6		8	5		3
	9	4			1	6		2
5		8	9			7	1	
6							3	
	7		1	3				
		3	4	6		2	7	

Puzzle #88 - Easy

	7		8	3				9
		3		6		8	7	4
6						5	2	
3		7			4	1		
		2		1		7	5	6
			7				3	2
	1	4				9	6	
	3	6		8	9			
				7	6		8	1

Puzzle #89 - Easy

	5			6	4		9	
8		6	7			5		1
		9			8			
	9	7	3				6	4
1				2	6	7		
				4				9
	1	8				9		7
			8		5	1	4	
3	7		4	1				

Puzzle #90 - Easy

2		9		4				
1	6		7	9	3			
		3	2			6		9
4		7	8	3		9		2
	9	1	5	2		4		8
8	3					5	9	1
	4	2						6
		5	3	8		2		

Puzzle #91 - Easy

	3			7		8		4
		6		5			3	9
		1	4			7	5	
		2		3			1	7
		4	5			9	6	
	9			6		3		2
		3	7	4		6	8	
7					5			
	4	9		8		2		5

Puzzle #92 - Easy

			6		2			
	1		9	3	7	6		8
		7					4	2
2		3	4	7	9		8	
			8		6			
	8	1						6
3		8	1	9		7		4
1						8		
9		6		2	8	5		1

Puzzle #93 - Easy

	1	8				6	7	
			6		3	9	8	
9		6	4		1			
1			7	3		4		
	2	3						7
7	6	5	2				1	
5		2		6				
	9				7		3	8
8	4	7	3				6	

Puzzle #94 - Easy

9		2		4				1
8			5				2	
		5	3		1			9
2				3		7	6	
7	5		9					8
	4			7	5		3	
	7			1				3
	2	1	4				9	
		9	2			1		7

Puzzle #95 - Easy

	3				6	7	8	4
		7		8	3			9
6						2	5	
			6		7	8		1
	4	1				6	9	
	6	3	9		8			
				7		3		2
	2				1	5	7	6
3	7		4				1	

Puzzle #96 - Easy

5			7	1				9
	6	9		8				7
	8		3			1		
4		8			5	6		
	7		4		8			3
6			1			2	4	
	1			7			9	4
	5			9	1	7		
9					4			6

Puzzle #97 - Easy

				9	8			
3	1			4				6
	4	5	2				3	7
5			6	8	9	7	2	
		2	4	5		8	6	3
						6		2
6	5		1		3		9	
	9	1			4	3		

Puzzle #98 - Easy

		6	2		4			1
	8	4	6			5		
7				3		8		4
6	9			7			8	
8			1					3
		5		9			1	7
1				4	9		7	
5			7			1	9	
		9		6		4		

Puzzle #99 - Easy

3	9		2	5		7		1
		6	4		3			9
	2	1			8	4		
6				2	5	9		4
9			6		1	2		8
					9			
		3						
	4	9		8		3		2
2		7		3		8		5

Puzzle #100 - Easy

			4		6	9	7	
		9	7	8			4	2
7						8	5	
4	2					1		
	7	5	3	4				6
9	1			6	5			
		2				4	6	
			8	3	9			
5	8							9

MEDIUM

Puzzle #1 - Medium

	8	7		4				
	9				2			
5		4		7	3	8		
	4	6	5					2
9	2				8	3		
3		1	2			5		
7	1						5	
	3							7
4		8	3				6	9

Puzzle #2 - Medium

	3				5	2		
		6	1	9				7
9		7						
	4				9	7		
3		1	5				6	
			4	6				
	6	9	3		2		1	5
5		8						3
			6	5			2	

Puzzle #3 - Medium

			4		1			2
4			7	6				
			8					
		3		4	6			1
1					9	6		
		6		5	8		9	4
		9		3				6
5				8	4	2		
3	6			1	7	5		

Puzzle #4 - Medium

				3			7	
		3	2		4		9	6
					7			8
7	9		6		8	3		
4			3					
	5			9				
5	8			4				
				2			4	9
6			7		3			2

Puzzle #5 - Medium

			4	6				
7					9			4
		6	5			1	3	
		2	6	5				
	5	1	3		2	9		6
	3					8	5	
2					5			3
						7	9	
	7		1	9		6		

Puzzle #6 - Medium

	6	2			7			
7		4	9		6			
8					3		7	5
6		7						1
	8	1					2	6
	3		6		9			7
			3					2
		3	7				4	
					4		3	

Puzzle #7 - Medium

		2	6	4				5
5			1		3			2
3				2	9	8		
8			4		5	3	7	
				9		2		
			7	8			4	
	5			1	7			
		7		3				
	6	9	8		4			3

Puzzle #8 - Medium

	6			2		7	3	
8	5							4
				9	4			2
9	7		3			6	8	
5								9
	4					3		
					7			3
		3		6	9	2	4	
				8			7	

Puzzle #9 - Medium

	5				2	6	1	7
	7		4	3		2		
6	3	7		4				9
9			7		3			6
7	8						6	
4		2	3			1	7	
		6				8		3

Puzzle #10 - Medium

	2		1	3				5
	5		6		4	2		
		8		9	2			3
		2			9			
7		3	4	5				8
4			7		8			
	3		8	4		9	6	
				7	1		5	
					3	7		

Puzzle #11 - Medium

					4			6
				5		2		
	6	8		1				
7	2					9		
				2		8		
					5			3
1	3			4				9
5	8	9		6	2	7		4
	7	6			3	5		

Puzzle #12 - Medium

	3				6	9		4
8		9		2			5	7
	5				4		3	2
2			1	5		4		6
			8				6	9
		2	6			3	7	8
		7				1		5

Puzzle #13 - Medium

5			1	3				6
4	6							
		9			4	7		
6	5							2
			8	5			3	
3		2	9		6		5	1
		5			3	2		
1	9		6				7	
			7	9				

Puzzle #14 - Medium

	3			7	1		4	2
			3		8			6
				6		8	7	
3	7		6				9	
		4	9			3	6	7
2			7	1	6	5		
	4	3			2	7		

Puzzle #15 - Medium

	2	6				8	1	
		7	9		6	3		
		1					7	6
			7			6	2	
	7	5	3					8
			6		9		4	7
	4				7		3	
	3		4					
		2			3			

Puzzle #16 - Medium

6	2		5	9	8	7	4	
	3			6	7	5		
4			1		3		9	
	5						3	
			7		2	9		
2						8		
	4						6	
5						2		
1				8	6			

Puzzle #17 - Medium

		4			9	3		1
	2	6		7	4	8	9	5
	3			5		7	6	
				9		2		7
		2		8				
	5				3			
		1				6	8	
	4				6			
		5		2				

Puzzle #18 - Medium

3	5				1		4	
6								
		9	3	6				
7	4		6	8	9			1
						8	7	4
1	8	3	4	5			6	
5	2				6			
		6	1	4				2
				9				

Puzzle #19 - Medium

7			5		1			
2			8	7	3	6		
			9	6		8		
9		8	7	5			2	
	3		4		9			6
		2	6		4	1	5	
	5		2	3				4

Puzzle #20 - Medium

5		7	2			8	9	
	9	4			6			3
	1	5					7	
7	3	8		6			2	
6		9		8				
3		2			4			5
	4	6	5	1		2		

Puzzle #21 - Medium

6	7	1		5			2	
2				7		4		3
8	3		6					
		6		8	7			
1		7	2		4	3		
	9		7	3	6			4
	6				9	7	3	

Puzzle #22 - Medium

1							5	
4							3	
	9		7	1		8		
		6		2	8	5		
				9			6	8
		2	6	7		3		4
	7		4		2			5
6		5	8					
	2	4	1	5				3

Puzzle #23 - Medium

		6	8	3		1	7	2
7			6				3	
9					7	6	8	
1	5	4	7	2			6	
		9		6				8
	3	8			5			7
4		7						
			1	9				
							2	5

Puzzle #24 - Medium

			8				3	5
	9	7				2		
5	6							
			7	4				
	3					5		2
			3		2		8	
	8		4	7		6		1
1		3		8	9	4	2	
7	4		5				9	3

Puzzle #25 - Medium

7		3		6			2	
	4		8	5				
	2						9	4
3				4				
	9		5					
6		8	9	7		3		
2		4			3		6	9
		7					8	
	3							7

Puzzle #26 - Medium

2	9			8	6			
						3		
	4		7		9			
		8				9	5	
					3			
6		5				7		4
	2	4	3				9	
7					2	6		3
3				7	4	8		

Puzzle #27 - Medium

	4			9		7	3	6
3		7		6				9
2			1	7	6		5	
	3	4			2		7	
			6				8	7
		3	7		1	2		4
				3	8	6		

Puzzle #28 - Medium

1		4		2		6		
		7		8			4	
8					5	3		
			8	5	1	2		
				9				6
2		8						1
			9			4		
7		2	5					
				4		1	2	8

Puzzle #29 - Medium

		7		5				
3			6		2	9		
8	6				7	1		
	7	9			1			4
6			9	8	4			7
				3	5			
2			8	7			5	
1		6						
7	3	8			6		2	

Puzzle #30 - Medium

	5		3	1		6		
6	4							
		9			4		7	
			9	7				
9	1			6				7
		5			3		2	
	3	2		9	6	1		5
			5	8				3
5	6					2		

Puzzle #31 - Medium

					1		5	
		4	9		5	2		8
9	5				8			
	7			2		1	8	
	2			8		4		7
4		1			2	6	3	
		2						4
		8	6	1				

Puzzle #32 - Medium

8	9		1	3			2	4
		5	7		4	3	9	
7		4			8	1		6
	2	3					8	
4		7						
					3	2		5
			5		6			
		8				5	3	
				7	9			2

Puzzle #33 - Medium

				7	2	9		
2	6		5		4			
			6				1	4
	8			2				
7	2	9			5	1		
6			8	4	1	7		
3	5					8		
		6					5	3
4		8		5	3			

Puzzle #34 - Medium

		2	4	1				
			8					
			7		6		4	
		1		6	4	3		
6				9			1	
	9	4		8	5	6		
		6			3	9		
2				4	8		5	
5				7	1		3	6

Puzzle #35 - Medium

1	2				4	8	9	
8				3				5
	7				5		1	
		7	8			1		
6				1				7
5		8	3		7	4		
7	5					9		
4		6			8			
				9				6

Puzzle #36 - Medium

	7		8	3				5
	8		9			6		
		6	4	5	1	2	7	
6		8			9			7
1	2	7	6			3	8	
		3			7		6	
	5	2						
			7		4			
						9	1	

Puzzle #37 - Medium

3		6	7		1	5		
	9				3			6
5			4		8	2		
4				7	6			
				8				
			1	4				2
	3		6		4			1
	6		8		5		9	4
1			9			6		

Puzzle #38 - Medium

		5		3		6		7
9					4		1	3
4		7		2	6	9	5	8
		9					7	2
3				5				
		8			2			
		2			5			
6				4				
					1	8		6

Puzzle #39 - Medium

7	1	2	6			8		3
8	6				9		7	
3					7	6		
			7		4			
2		5						
						1		9
		8	9					6
6			4	5	1	7		2
		7	8	3			5	

Puzzle #40 - Medium

		6			5		7	
	9		8			4		1
			9	1				
	5		2	7				
4	7		1		8	5	6	
6						8		7
						3		8
		9			3		1	
8			4	5		7		

Puzzle #41 - Medium

		2			5	7	1	6
3	4				7			2
4			7	6	3	9		
	7	3		9		6		
				7	8		6	
			6			3		8
	3		2	4			7	1

Puzzle #42 - Medium

		6					3	8
7	8					6		
4		2			3	7		1
	7			3	4			2
	5		2			1	7	6
9			3		7		6	
6	3	7		4			9	

Puzzle #43 - Medium

2	4		3					9
		3		7	4	8		
		7			2	6	3	
						3		
4			7		9			
9		2		8	6			
	8					9		5
					3			
	5	6				7	4	

Puzzle #44 - Medium

2			8		4			5
5			1		7	6		3
	6		3				9	
	2			4	1			
				8				
			6	7				4
	1		4		6		3	
	4	9	5		8		6	
6					9			1

Puzzle #45 - Medium

8	6		7				9	
3					6		7	
7	1	2		3	8			6
				9	1			
2		5						
							4	7
		7	5			3		8
6				2	7	5	1	4
		8		6				9

Puzzle #46 - Medium

		5			2	8	7	
			6		1			
		2	8	3	7			6
1				6	8			7
			7				5	
9					3	6		2
	7				6	9	8	4
							3	5
	4		9	7				1

Puzzle #47 - Medium

2			6	3		7		
4		7	8			3		
	3				9		2	4
			3					
9	7						4	
6		8				2	9	
			9		5			8
			7	4		6		5
3								

Puzzle #48 - Medium

		3					5	2
			2	3		8		
				7	4			
7		4		5		9		3
1	3		9		8	2	4	
		8		4	7		6	1
				8		3		5
5		6						
	7	9					2	

Puzzle #49 - Medium

		8			7			
	9	6		2	4		3	
	7		3					
3				6	8	9		7
			9			5		
				3				4
			4			8		5
		2		7	3			6
	4	9	2					

Puzzle #50 - Medium

8			4		7		2	
2			1	8			7	
	8						5	9
	1			5				
	5	9	2		8	4		
1		6				8		
	2		6	3		1		4
					4	2		

Puzzle #51 - Medium

	7	6	4					
1	4					2		
	8							
9			1				6	
6		4		3		1		
8		5		6		4		9
4		8	5				2	
		3		9		6		
7		1	3		6		5	

Puzzle #52 - Medium

			4		1			2
			8					
4			7	6				
5				8	4	2		
		9		3				6
3	6			1	7	5		
1					9	6		
		6		5	8		9	4
		3		4	6			1

Puzzle #53 - Medium

	9				5			
8		6		7	9		3	
		3		4				
7								8
4		2	3			9		6
	3					7		
	2					4		9
	4			5	8			
3		7		6				2

Puzzle #54 - Medium

6		9	4		8			3
5			7	1				
		7		3				
	3		9	2		8		
	5		3		1			2
		2		4	6			5
				9		2		
	8		5		4	3	7	
				8	7		4	

Puzzle #55 - Medium

4	6					8		
			6				9	
7		5		9				
5	8			4		7		3
6			7				1	
	7			1				8
		7			1	5		
8			5				3	
1		2		8	9	4		

Puzzle #56 - Medium

5				2	4		7	
3			5		1		2	4
					8	6		5
		5	2	8				6
4		3	7		6			2
8	6		9					
		8	1		7		9	
	3					4		
	5					1		

Puzzle #57 - Medium

9					5	6		
	5		2				9	
1			3		6	4		5
	3		6				4	
		9		5				3
6		7	9	8				1
7			5	3				
	2						7	
			1		2			6

Puzzle #58 - Medium

		7	6				3	
	6		8	3		1	7	2
		9			7	6	8	
	7	4						
							2	5
			1	9				
3	8				5			7
5	4	1	7	2			6	
	9			6				8

Puzzle #59 - Medium

	8		5	6				
	1	5	4		2			3
2	4				7			5
				1			5	
				4			3	
	7	1			9	8		
		9					6	8
	6	7	2			3		4
8		2	6			5		

Puzzle #60 - Medium

		7	6		9		3	
	2	6				1	8	
		1				7		6
			9		6	4		7
					7	2	6	
	7	5			3			8
		2	3					
	3				4			
	4		7			3		

Puzzle #61 - Medium

			5					3
7	2						9	
					2		8	
					5		2	
	6	8			1			
			4					6
1	3				4			9
	7	6	3				5	
5	8	9	2		6		7	4

Puzzle #62 - Medium

	2			8	9	5	7	
		6	3				4	9
		4	5			3	2	
1	5			2			6	4
6					2	7	8	3
					7		5	1
8						6	9	

Puzzle #63 - Medium

5				9		2		
	1		4		5	3	6	
	9		6				5	
	6	7			1	9		8
3				4		6		
		9			3			5
	7					5		3
2				7				
					6	1	2	

Puzzle #64 - Medium

				6	7		1	
			8		1		6	2
9		6	3				7	
4								3
		7			3			4
		3					2	
7			6		2			
6		9		7	4			
3				8			5	7

Puzzle #65 - Medium

9	8	6	1				7	4
			4	8	7			
	5	4			6	3	1	8
1					4		3	5
	6	3				9		
							6	
	9							
6							5	2
	4	1	2			6		

Puzzle #66 - Medium

1	5	8					2	
			8		2			1
	9							6
	4					2	1	8
		5	2		7			
		9					4	
	2		4		1		6	
5					8		3	
	8		7			4		

Puzzle #67 - Medium

				7	2		5	
	5	6	8		1		7	4
7	8							6
1	4				8		9	
				1	9			
		7	5			6		
	7			5	4			8
8	3							
		1	3			9		

Puzzle #68 - Medium

			7		8		4	
					9			2
		8	4	5			7	3
2			6		4	5		
		5	1	3		2		
		3		9	2			8
7					3			
9	6		8	4		3		
	5			7	1			

Puzzle #69 - Medium

		6		2		7	3	8
		8				6		9
				7			1	5
	2		8	9		5		7
6					3		9	4
4					5	3		2
	5	1	2				4	6

Puzzle #70 - Medium

2						4		9
4				5	8			
	3	7		6				2
3						7		
	4	2	3			9		6
	7							8
9					5			
	8	6		7	9		3	
		3		4				

Puzzle #71 - Medium

	6	4	1					3
	8	5	4		9			6
	9			6		1		
7		6				4		
4	1		2					
8								
		3	6					9
	7	1		5		3	6	
	4	8		2		5		

Puzzle #72 - Medium

5				2		6	1	7
7			3		4	2		
8	7						6	
	4	2			3	1	7	
		6				8		3
	9			3	7			6
3	6	7	4					9

Puzzle #73 - Medium

7		3			2	6		
	2			4	9			
	4					5	8	
3						4		
6		8	3			7	9	
	9						5	
		7			8			
	3			7				
2		4		9	6			3

Puzzle #74 - Medium

3					2			
		4	3					
7			4			3		
			2		6	1		8
6		9			7			3
					1	7	6	
9		6				4	7	
		3	7		5		8	
		7				2		6

Puzzle #75 - Medium

8		1			2			7
	7	4			8			2
				8		9		5
	8	2	9	5			4	
5				1				
3		6		2		4	1	
	4						2	
			6		1		8	

Puzzle #76 - Medium

		2					9	
4						7	8	
7		3	8			4		5
	2		5			1		3
	5				2	6	4	
		8	3				2	9
				5			1	7
	3			6	9	8		4
					7		3	

Puzzle #77 - Medium

	5	8	3		7		4	
	6			1		7		
		7	8				1	
	4	6			8			
				9		6		
5	7						9	
	8			3		5		
7					5			1
2	1				4		8	9

Puzzle #78 - Medium

		8						
	6	7						4
1		4			2			
4	8		2					5
	3				6		9	
7	1		5			6		3
6	4				1		3	
8	5			9	4		6	
9			6					1

Puzzle #79 - Medium

8								
7	6							4
4		1			2			
	1	7	5			6		3
	8	4	2					5
	3				6		9	
		9	6					1
	5	8		9	4		6	
	4	6			1		3	

Puzzle #80- Medium

		7		3			6	9
		1	7		6			
	2	6	1	8				
			4		7		9	6
	7	5			8			3
			2	6				7
		2					3	
	4		3				7	
	3							4

Puzzle #81 - Medium

		6	4	8	9			7
7	9		1					4
			5	3				
6		8	7				1	
	7			5				
		3	2		6		9	
3	8	7	6			2		
	6	1						
		2		7	8	5		

Puzzle #82 - Medium

								3
5	9				8			
	7	4	6		5			
	8		3			7		4
	6	3	7					2
9				2	4		3	
			2	9		8		6
	3							
				4			7	9

Puzzle #83 - Medium

2	7						5	
				4			9	
			2	1	8			4
7			4					8
4	1			6				2
	8			3		5		
					6			9
				2		1	8	5
8	2				1			

Puzzle #84 - Medium

	3							4
	5							1
8			7		1		9	
3		4	6		7	2		
5				8	2	6		
	6	8			9			
		3	1		5	4	2	
			8			5		6
		5	4	2			7	

Puzzle #85 - Medium

	2							8
1	4	8	7				6	
5			1			9	7	2
4		5					2	6
2	7		9					
		6		4	1			
3	5					8	4	
			8				3	5
				3	5	6		

Puzzle #86 - Medium

			8	6			9	
	6				5	8	2	
	2		4		3		7	6
2	4		3				5	1
7			5			2		4
	5	6						8
		4		3				
		1		5				
9					8		1	7

Puzzle #87 - Medium

4			3		1		9	
	3		7	6				5
6	2		8	9	5		4	7
	5						3	
2								8
			2		7			9
1			6	8				
	4						6	
5								2

Puzzle #88 - Medium

6		7			1			
	8	1	2		6			
	3				7		9	6
		3	4					7
			3				4	
					2			3
	6	2					7	
8			7		5		3	
7		4					6	9

Puzzle #89 - Medium

9					5			2
		6		9			5	
	5	4		1			6	3
4					3			6
	1		7	6		8		9
	3		9			5		
7					2			
	6						2	1
				7		3		5

Puzzle #90 - Medium

		6	7		3			2
				2			4	9
	8	5		4				
					7			8
3			2		4		9	6
				3			7	
	9	7	6		8	3		
	5			9				
		4	3					

Puzzle #91 - Medium

	4		6	3	7		9	
3		7	9				6	
2				5		1	7	6
	3	4		7				2
		3	4		2	7		1
			7	8		6		
					6		3	8

Puzzle #92 - Medium

					8			7
3			9		6		2	4
			7			3		
		5				9		
	4						3	
	7	9		3			6	8
	6				2		7	3
	5	8				4		
			4		9	2		

Puzzle #93 - Medium

	3	2	5			4		
4		6		2			1	5
9		4	3			6		
	5	7		8	9			2
	6	9					8	
1		5			7			
3	7	8			2		6	

Puzzle #94 - Medium

					8	6	5	
	3			5	1		4	2
	5		2		4			7
	8	6		9				
5			8	2			6	
3	4			7	6		2	
		3				4		
8				1	7			9
		5				1		

Puzzle #95 - Medium

1	3			6		5		
						4		6
		4			7		9	
6			7			1		9
7	9							
		3			2		5	
8	5		3					
				2		6		5
9		6	5	1		3	2	

Puzzle #96 - Medium

9						5		7
				8			6	4
	6		9					
	7		1					6
1					8		7	
4				7	3		8	5
	5		3					8
		1		5		7		
8		9		4		2		1

Puzzle #97 - Medium

3	2		5			4		
	6	4		2			5	1
6	9							8
	5	1			7			
7	8	3			2			6
5	7			8	9		2	
	4	9	3			6		

Puzzle #98 - Medium

6		9	5	1		2	3	
				2			6	5
	5	8	3					
	9	7						
3					2	5		
		6	7				1	9
							4	6
	3	1		6			5	
4					7	9		

Puzzle #99 - Medium

7		5		2			8	9
4	9				6	3		
5	1							7
9		6	8					
8	3	7	6					2
6	4		1	5			2	
2		3			4	5		

Puzzle #100 - Medium

	3			6	9		4	8
				5		1	7	
					7	3		
3		7	8				5	4
		4				8		7
2						9		
	2		5				3	1
8			3			2	9	
	5				2	4		6

Puzzle #101 - Medium

2				6		7	3	
9		4						2
			8	5				4
		7						3
8							7	
6		9			3	2	4	
				4		3		
			5					9
	3		9	7		6	8	

Puzzle #102 - Medium

3	5						4	8
					8	5	3	
			5	3				6
4		5				6	2	
2	7				9			
		6	1	4				
1	4	8			7		6	
5					1	2	7	9
	2					8		

Puzzle #103 - Medium

8			3	5				
			4		8	5		3
	3	5			6			
1			7	2	9			5
7			6			4	8	1
				8		2		
	4	1					6	
			2	6			5	4
9						7		2

Puzzle #104 - Medium

5					6			9
		2	9			5		
6		3		5	4			1
			7			2		
2		1		6				
	3	5						7
	8	9		1			7	6
	5			3			9	
		6	4			3		

Puzzle #105 - Medium

8		9	4				2	1
	5			3				8
		1	5				7	
	6			9				
9							5	7
			8			6		4
	7			1				6
1					8	7		
4			7		3	8		5

Puzzle #106 - Medium

6	3		2					7
8			4	7				3
		9			3	2	4	
3								
			6	8		9		2
			9		7	4		
			3					
9		5					8	
7	4						5	6

Puzzle #107 - Medium

	2					6	5	
3				8	5			
5	1		6	9		3		2
						4	6	
	6			1	3	5		
		7	4					9
		2	3					5
				7	9			
7				6		1	9	

Puzzle #108 - Medium

	9		6			8		
	8	3			5	7		
1	4	5	2	7				6
	6		3	8		2	1	7
7				6				3
9					7		6	8
						5		2
4	7							
			9	1				

Puzzle #109 - Medium

		4						3
9				7	1		8	
		1						5
2	4			1	5	3		
7			2	4		5		
	5	6		8				
					9	8		6
	2			6	7	4	3	
	6		8		2		5	

Puzzle #110 - Medium

		9			5	6		
		1	3		6	4	5	
5			2					9
2								7
			1		2		6	
		7	5	3				
	7	6	9	8			1	
3			6					4
	9			5			3	

Puzzle #111 - Medium

	5				1	9	7	2
		2						8
8	1	4			7		6	
6			1	4				
	2	7			9			
5	4						2	6
			5	3		6		
	3	5				8	4	
					8		3	5

Puzzle #112 - Medium

		3		5			6	7
	6	2		7	4	5	9	8
	4				9	1		3
	1						8	6
	5			2				
		4			6			
		5			3			
				9		7		2
	2			8				

Puzzle #113 - Medium

				8		5	9	
		5		1				
2	8		9	5				4
6		3		2			4	1
			6		1			8
	4							2
4	7				8	2		
1		8			2	7		

Puzzle #114 - Medium

		2	8		9	7	5	
	6			3		4		9
	4			5		2	3	
1		5	2			6		4
					7	5		1
8						9	6	
6					2	8	7	3

Puzzle #115 - Medium

9	3		5			7	4	
	1	6	4	7			8	
2		4		8	9	1		3
		2					9	7
						5	6	
3	5		8					
			7	4				
	2	5					3	
8			3		2			

Puzzle #116 - Medium

2			7		4	8		
7				8	1	2		
		8				1		6
		2	4					
	4	1		3	6		2	
				5			1	
5	9						8	
		4	8		2		5	9

Puzzle #117 - Medium

5		1						7
8	7	3		6				2
9	6			8				
6		4		1	5		2	
2	3		4			5		
7	5				2		8	9
4		9	6			3		

Puzzle #118 - Medium

			5	3		8		
7	9				2			
	6	5						
	4	7	3	9		5		
3		1		2	4		8	9
	8		1		6	4	7	
						7	4	
				8		3		2
	3		2		5			

Puzzle #119 - Medium

8	9	5		7	4		6	2
7	6			5				3
3		1			9		4	
				8			2	
2		7		9				
					3			5
				2			5	
6	8						1	
					6			4

Puzzle #120 - Medium

	8	9		2		7	5	
3					6	4		9
	2		1	5		6		4
5					4	2	3	
		2	6			8	7	3
		7				5		1
			8			9	6	

Puzzle #121 - Medium

8	6				1			
					5	2		
			4				6	
9	8	5	2		6	7	4	
6	7		3			5		
	3	1			4		9	
	2	7				9		
			5				3	
					2	8		

Puzzle #122 - Medium

		8	2			7	4	
		2	7				1	8
	6	1		8				
				2		4		
2				1	4		6	3
8			5		9			
5	9			4		8	2	
1								5

Puzzle #123 - Medium

3					4			
		8		9		1	7	
5					1			
	4	3	2			7	6	
		5	6			2		8
6	8					9		
	5			7			4	2
			5		6		8	
	3		4	2		5	1	

Puzzle #124 - Medium

5					1			
					8		5	9
	2	8	9		5	4		
	4	7		8			2	
8	1			2			7	
		4				2		
			6	1		8		
3	6				2	1		4

Puzzle #125 - Medium

	2		8					
5					3			
			9			7	2	
2	6		7		4	5	8	9
3			5				7	6
	4				9	1	3	
	5		2					
4					6			
	1						6	8

Puzzle #126 - Medium

	3		9	6		7		
1	8					6		2
7		6				1		
			4					3
				3		2		
3				7				4
4		7	6	9				
		8	3			5		7
2	6		7					

Puzzle #127 - Medium

6			5	2				
	9							
	4	1			6		2	
1			3	5		4		
	6	3			9			
			6					
						7	4	8
9	8	6	7	4			1	
	5	4	1	8	3	6		

Puzzle #128 - Medium

		5		7				
	7		8		6			1
6	2		3					9
	1			9	7		4	
	5	3						
9	4	8	6				7	
	6		7	8	3	2		
8		7	2			5		
			1	6				

Puzzle #129 - Medium

		3	5				8	
		6			2	4	1	
	4				8	7		
		2	1	8	5			
6					9			
1						8	2	
		4		9				
8	2	1			4			
				5		2	7	

Puzzle #130 - Medium

	6	5				8		
7					5	4	2	
2		4			3	1		5
				6	8			9
		2	3		4	6		7
		6	5				8	2
	4			3				
	1			5				
9			8			7		1

Puzzle #131 - Medium

4		2		5	1			3
5	6				8			
		7	2		4			5
	4						3	
	1						5	
		9		1	7	8		
				9			6	8
6			8	2		5		
2				7	6	3		4

Puzzle #132 - Medium

8		5				4		
			4	9		2		
		6		2			7	3
9		7			3		6	8
5						9		
		4					3	
			7			3		
	3		9	6			2	4
				8				7

Puzzle #133 - Medium

	7	9					2	
5		6						
					8	3		5
		3					5	2
			4		7			
				2	3	8		
1	3		8	9		2	4	
		8	7		4		6	1
7		4			5	9		3

Puzzle #134 - Medium

	9					6		8
	7	6			2		3	4
8	2				6		5	
	1	7		9			8	
			1			5		
			4			3		
	5	1		2	4			3
2		4		7				5
		8	6		5			

Puzzle #135 - Medium

	4		9				7	
3		1			5	6		
				6	4			
5		8						3
				5	6	2		
	6	9	2		3	1		5
9		7						
	3		5				2	
		6		9	1			7

Puzzle #136 - Medium

					6			
	1		5		3			4
6		3		9				
4		1		6			2	
	6		2		5			
9								
8	9	6	4		7		1	
5		4	8	3	1			6
						8	4	7

Puzzle #137 - Medium

			8		3			
5	4				7		8	
		3		1				9
7	2					5		
	1	8		6	5	7	4	
			7		8		6	
		5		7				6
	8		1		4	9		
1	9							

Puzzle #138 - Medium

4			3	7		5		8
	7				1	6		
1			8					7
	5				3	8		
		1		5			7	
8		9		4		1	2	
	6				9			
				8		4		6
9						7	5	

Puzzle #139 - Medium

	6		5		3			
5		3		8				
	8	4					5	3
		6		7		8	4	1
8							2	
2	9	7		1				5
6		2				5		4
			1		4	6		
				9			7	2

Puzzle #140 - Medium

	6		7	8				
3		8			6			
	7	1	4		2	3		
		2		7		4	3	
7	1	6		5				2
6			9			7		3
9			6	3	7		4	

Puzzle #141 - Medium

		6		9		8		
7		2	1	4	5			6
	5			8	3	7		
1		9						
						5		2
			4	7				
	7		9				6	8
6			7					3
8		3		6		2	1	7

Puzzle #142 - Medium

9	4			3			6	
	7	5	8		9			2
4	6		2			1		5
	2	3		5			4	
	9	6				8		
3	8	7			2	6		
1	5				7			

Puzzle #143 - Medium

	3		9		6	4	2	
			7					3
					8	7		
		5						9
4							3	
7		9		3		8	6	
5		8						4
			4		9			2
6					2	3	7	

Puzzle #144 - Medium

		5			2			9
	9		5			6		
	1		6		3	4	5	
7	6			8	9		1	
9				5			3	
		3			6			4
	7			3	5			
		2						7
			2		1		6	

Puzzle #145 - Medium

6	7		2				3	4
	2	8	6				5	
	9					6		8
				4		3		
7	1				9		8	
				1		5		
4		2			7			5
1	5		4		2			3
8			5	6				

Puzzle #146 - Medium

3		7		6		2		
	4			5	8			
	2					9		4
4		2	3			6		9
7						8		
	3							7
		3		4				
8		6		7	9		3	
	9				5			

Puzzle #147 - Medium

			8	3		6		
					6		8	7
		3	1		7	2		4
	2		6	7	1		5	
3		4	2				7	
	3	7		6				9
4				9		7	3	6

Puzzle #148 - Medium

9				8			6	
4	1	5			6	7	2	
8		3		7				5
6			1	2	7	8	3	
	7				3	6		
	9		6		8			7
				5	2			
7	4							
						1	9	

Puzzle #149 - Medium

		3				4		
9							5	
	8	6			3	7	9	
	7		8					
3				7				
	4	2	6	9				3
4						5	8	
	3	7	2			6		
2			9	4				

Puzzle #150 - Medium

2			8		4			5
5			1		7		6	3
	6		3			9		
6					9			1
	4	9	5		8	6		
	1		4		6	3		
				8				
			6	7				4
	2			4	1			

Puzzle #151 - Medium

				4			5	8
2			7		3		6	
9		4		2				
6		9	2		4	3		
		7		3				
8					7			
	3		6		8		7	9
			3				4	
				9				5

Puzzle #152 - Medium

2	6		7	4		9	8	5
	4			9			3	1
3			5			6	7	
	5		2					
	1					8	6	
4				6				
	2		8					
5				3				
			9				2	7

Puzzle #153 - Medium

	6			3		9	4	
2			8		9		7	5
					7	1	5	
		8					9	6
		6			2	3	8	7
5		1	2			4	6	
	4			5			2	3

Puzzle #154 - Medium

			4					3
					3	2		
	3				7			4
	2	6	7					
8			3			5		7
7	4		6		9			
	1	8				6		2
6	7					1		
		3	9		6	7		

Puzzle #155 - Medium

		6					4	
2								5
			6	8				1
9			2		7			
8								2
		3					5	
5			7	6			3	
7		4	8	9	5		2	6
		9	3		1			4

Puzzle #156 - Medium

				7		3		5
		7	2					
6							2	1
	6			9			5	
5	4			1			6	3
		9	5					2
		4	3					6
3					9	5		
1				6	7	8		9

Puzzle #157 - Medium

	7	4			8			3
		2	3		6			7
3				9		2	4	
				5	9		8	
		3						
			4		7		5	6
	8	6				9		2
					3			
7		9				4		

Puzzle #158 - Medium

					6	8		7
2		7	5					
1	8		7		4	5	6	
4		5			8	7		
						3		8
	3			9			1	
8			9			4		1
	5			6			7	
9		1						

Puzzle #159 - Medium

		6		3			9	
2				8	4	5		
5				1	7	3		6
6					9	1		
	9	4		5	8		6	
		1		4	6		3	
			8					
			7	6		4		
		2	4		1			

Puzzle #160 - Medium

	7	5	8		9			2
9	4			3			6	
3	8	7			2	6		
	9	6				8		
1	5				7			
	2	3		5			4	
4	6		2			1		5

Puzzle #161 - Medium

	3	6		5		7		1
9			6					3
	5			2		4		8
			2			1	4	
	4						7	6
							8	
6			4		9	8		5
3			1			6		4
	1			6		9		

Puzzle #162 - Medium

		4	9			3	1	
3				5		7		6
2		6	4	7		8	5	9
		2		8				
5			3					
				9		2	7	
		5		2				
		1				6		8
4			6					

Puzzle #163 - Medium

6			1	2	7		3	8
	7				3			6
	9		6		8	7		
				5	2			
7	4							
							9	1
4	1	5			6		2	7
9				8			6	
8		3		7		5		

Puzzle #164 - Medium

	3			4				6
6		7	1			8		9
		9	3			5		
	2			7				
7						3		5
			6				2	1
9					6		5	
1			5		4		6	3
	5			9				2

Puzzle #165 - Medium

7				2	6			
3			8				5	7
6		9	7	4				
9		6			3		7	
				1	8		6	2
			6	7			1	
		3					2	
4								3
		7		3				4

Puzzle #166 - Medium

	6			8	3			
4	2		7	1				3
7		8	6					
6	7	3			9	4		
9					6		3	7
		5	1	6	7		2	
		7		2		3		4

Puzzle #167 - Medium

7				5		2	4	
2		4		3			1	5
	6	5					8	
		6			5	8		2
			6	8				9
		2		4	3		6	7
	4		3					
9					8		7	1
	1		5					

Puzzle #168 - Medium

6		8			1		7	
	7							5
		3			9	6	2	
	6	1						
3	8	7	2				6	
		2	5			8		7
		6		7		9	4	8
7	9			4			1	
							5	3

Puzzle #169 - Medium

4		9						2
		2		6		3	7	
			8	5				4
				4			3	
			5					9
	3		9	7		8	6	
9		6			3	4	2	
		8				7		
7								3

Puzzle #170 - Medium

				8			5	3
			3		5	6		
3		5				8		4
2		7		9				
	6		4		1			
4	5						6	2
1	8	4		7				6
		2					8	
5				1		9	2	7

Puzzle #171 - Medium

	8	7					4	
5		4			8	3	7	
	9					2		
3		1			5			2
9	2				3	8		
	4	6	2					5
4		8	9	6				3
7	1			5				
	3		7					

Puzzle #172 - Medium

		3		6		4		
6	7			9	8			1
	9				5			3
		5		2		9		
1			6	3			4	5
9			5				6	
		2				7		
7				5	3			
			2	1				6

Puzzle #173 - Medium

	9		8				1	7
		4			3			
		1			5			
2			3	4			7	6
				8	6		9	
6			5			8	2	
4	2			3			5	1
5		6						8
	7			5		2		4

Puzzle #174 - Medium

5	4				7			8
		3	1				9	
				8	3			
1	9							
		5	7				6	
	8			1	4	9		
7	2					5		
	1	8	6		5	7		4
				7	8			6

Puzzle #175 - Medium

9	2		8					3
3		1			2			5
	4	6			5	2		
	8	7		4				
5		4	3	7				8
	9		2					
	3					7		
7	1						5	
4		8			3	9	6	

Puzzle #176 - Medium

4	1			2		3		6
	8		6		1			
	2						4	
	4		9	5			8	2
9		5		8				
				1		5		
		7			2	8		1
		2			8		7	4

Puzzle #177 - Medium

		8				5		6
5		1	3			4	2	
	2	4	5				7	
9			8	6				
2	8				5	6		
7		6	4		3	2		
1		7			8		9	
				3				4
				5				1

Puzzle #178 - Medium

	1			4		9		7
9	4	8		7			6	
	5	3						
		5				7		
6	2		9				3	
	7		1				8	6
8		7			5		2	
						6	1	
	6				2	8	7	3

Puzzle #179 - Medium

7		3	5	4				8
		2			9			
4				7	8			
		8	9		2			3
	5			6	4	2		
	2		3	1				5
			7		1		5	
	3		4	8		9	6	
					3	7		

Puzzle #180 - Medium

	6	4						
9				7				4
		5	6			1	3	
						7	9	
	9	1			7	6		
5				2				3
					3	8	5	
2		3	1		5	9		6
	5	6	2					

Puzzle #181 - Medium

5	8	1				2		
			2	8			1	
9							6	
	5		7	2				
	9					4		
4						1	8	2
2			1	4		6		
		5	8			3		
8				7				4

Puzzle #182 - Medium

			5	8	1		2	
			9					6
8		2						1
7			8			4		
		8			5		3	
4		1	2				6	
			4			2	1	8
2		7		5				
				9			4	

Puzzle #183 - Medium

8		9	7	6			1	
5			9				3	
		6			3	4		
	2	1					6	
					2	7		
3		5		7				
	6	3		1			5	4
	5			9				6
		2			5	9		

Puzzle #184 - Medium

	1			6		7		
7		3	8	5			4	
		8	7				1	
				7	5		9	
	9					6		
8			6	4				
	3			8		5		
5					7			1
4				1	2		8	9

Puzzle #185 - Medium

9	7		4					
6		8	9	2				
							3	
2				7		3	6	
	3		2		4			9
4		7		3			8	
3								
				6	5	4	7	
					8		9	5

Puzzle #186 - Medium

		8						
1		4				2		
	6	7			4			
9					1			6
8	5			6		4	9	
6	4			3		1		
7	1		6		3			5
	3			9		6		
4	8				5			2

Puzzle #187 - Medium

	1					7		6
	6	2				1	8	
	7		6		9		3	
					7	2	6	
	5	7			3			8
			9		6	4		7
		3			4			
		4	7			3		
	2		3					

Puzzle #188 - Medium

3			5				6	7
	4			9		1		3
2	6		7	4		5	9	8
	5		2					
4				6				
	1						8	6
			9			7		2
	2		8					
5				3				

Puzzle #189 - Medium

		3		2	5			
			8			3		2
						7	4	
	7	9			2			
			3	5		8		
5		6						
1	3		2		4		8	9
7		4	9	3		5		
		8		1	6	4	7	

Puzzle #190 - Medium

3	6	7	9				4	
	9		6			7		3
5			7	6	1			2
7				2		4	3	
8	7				6			
	4	2		1	7	3		
		6	3	8				

Puzzle #191 - Medium

8				2	9			3
	5		6	4		2		
	2		1		3			5
				3		7		
				1	7		5	
	3		8		4	9	6	
		4	7	8				
2				9				
3		7	4		5			8

Puzzle #192 - Medium

		3		6	9		2	4
					7	3		
				8				7
8	5					4		
	6			2			7	3
				9	4	2		
	4						3	
9	7		3				6	8
5						9		

Puzzle #193 - Medium

7			1	8	4			6
					2		8	
1			5			9	2	7
9			2		7			
	1	4		6				
			4	5			6	2
8							5	3
	5	3				6		
			3		5	8		4

Puzzle #194 - Medium

	5	2				6		
								9
6				2			1	4
	6							
	3	5	4			1		
9							3	6
	7	4		1		9	6	8
			7	4	8			
3	1	8	6				4	5

Puzzle #195 - Medium

	3		6		2	9		
	8	6			7	1		
7				5				
8	7	3			6			2
6	1							
	2		8	7				5
	6		9	8	4		7	
				3	5			
9		7			1		4	

Puzzle #196 - Medium

		9			6	5		
		1	5		4	6	3	
5				9			2	
2				7				
			6			2	1	
		7					5	3
3				4			6	
	9		3					5
	7	6	1				9	8

Puzzle #197 - Medium

	6	2	9	8	5	7	4	
		3	6	7		5		
	4			3	1		9	
		4					6	
	1		8	6				
	5					2		
		5					3	
	2					8		
				2	7	9		

Puzzle #198 - Medium

1			6	4				3
4	9		8	5				6
		6	9				1	
6				3				9
		2	4	8			5	
		5	7	1		6	3	
				6	7		4	
					8			
2			1		4			

Puzzle #199 - Medium

7	3		9				6	
		4	6	3	7		9	
					6	8	3	
3			4		2	1		7
			7	8				6
	2			5		6	7	1
4		3		7		2		

Puzzle #200 - Medium

		3			6		4	
6	7		8		9	1		
	9		5			3		
		5			2		9	
9				5				6
1				6	3	5		4
		2					7	
				2	1	6		
7			3		5			

HARD

Puzzle #1 - Hard

		8		9	1			
		6	8					9
9	7		5					
				2				7
		2			7	4	9	
	8			6		3		
	2		9			5	3	
4					8		2	
3								1

Puzzle #2 - Hard

	1						5	6
		5		1		7		
			2		3	8		
	8		1	3				
	2	3		9				
7					4			8
				8		9		5
1		6					8	
	7		5				4	

Puzzle #3 - Hard

			6			5		1
	2				3			
	9				1	3	6	
5					6			
				3		6		
	1	6		4	8		3	7
9		3		1				6
				7				8
8	5		2					

Puzzle #4 - Hard

	9	5					2	8
1	3					9	4	
4		1		8	7			
7	8		1		2			
		3	5			6		
			7		6	2		
			4			1	7	

Puzzle #5 - Hard

			2		3	5		
					5	4	8	
				7				1
	5		6					8
	2		1	9			6	
		4				7		
		2		4			5	
	7				2			
		6	7				3	4

Puzzle #6 - Hard

				7	1	9		2
			6	9			3	4
8		3	1		2			
4	1			3	8			
	6		7			5		
5	8					4		
	2					1		8

Puzzle #7 - Hard

1	6		8					
				9	5			8
		7	4				5	
		1	5		6			
	5			7				1
				8		3	2	
7					8	4		
	3	2						9
		8					1	3

Puzzle #8 - Hard

	7			4				
		5				8		1
	8		6			9		
	9		5	8		7	3	
		6		7	2			
7							6	5
3			2		9			
	6		4			5		
	1						4	

Puzzle #9 - Hard

			9	4			3	1
				2	8	5	9	
7		6	2					
4			1	7				
5			6			3		
	8	7				1		4
1		2					8	7

Puzzle #10 - Hard

			9			6		2
9				8	5			
		8	1				7	
	1			9				7
5						3	4	
3		2					9	
	3	4			9			
			8	6			2	
2					7	8		

Puzzle #11 - Hard

9		3	8					1
	4						3	
		1		5			2	
2		8		7		1		
	7				1			
3					6			5
	8		5			6		
				4	8	5		
			9				8	7

Puzzle #12 - Hard

		4						1
			9		2		3	
	5				4			6
			2	7		6		
	7	3		8	5			9
5		6					7	
1	8					5		
	9				6			8
				4				7

Puzzle #13 - Hard

				7				1
			5			8	4	
			3		2		5	
2				4		5		
6					7	3		4
	7		2					
	2			9	1	6		
	5				6			8
4							7	

Puzzle #14 - Hard

		4	3					
	1		2					5
9	3			1			8	
		7				1		
2	8				1			7
3				5		6		
					5	8		4
			8	7			9	
		8			6		5	

Puzzle #15 - Hard

	6				8			5
			7				4	
	1	9		6				2
3	2		5					
5			4	8				
		7			1			
	7			3	4		6	
		4		5			2	
2								7

Puzzle #16 - Hard

				3	5		6	
6	8				1	7		
				6		3		
		5	2	9		1		
3						6		
9		8						5
1	7					4	3	
			3	1		8		6
		2			6			

Puzzle #17 - Hard

				1	7	4		
				2		7		6
	3			6		5		
3		1		9	4			
9	5		8		2			
	1	4					8	7
8		7				1		2

Puzzle #18 - Hard

5					9		8	
	8	1		4				
	4			3				6
1				8			7	
	2				7	8		
			3		4		9	5
	6				8		1	
4			1			9		
8		9				3		

Puzzle #19 - Hard

5							9	8
	6						3	
	1			9	2			5
			6					2
	4	3				7	1	
6	8			1	3			
	3			6				
	7		1			8	6	
		6	5	3				

Puzzle #20 - Hard

		1			9	3		6
6						5	1	
		3			2			
	3					6		
	4	8		6	1		7	3
		6	5					
	7						8	
2			8		5			
	1		9	3			6	

Puzzle #21 - Hard

		3						
1						2	8	6
4		8					5	
8		2		1				
		1			6			7
3				7	9			
				2	4	8		
				9		1	4	5
					3			

Puzzle #22 - Hard

	3			5			6	
				7	6		2	
				4		7	1	
9	5					2		8
3		1				4	9	
8		7		1	2			
	1	4	8		7			

Puzzle #23 - Hard

	8	4						5
		1				6	2	8
	3							
			3					
			4		2		8	
					9	5	1	4
	2	8			1			
		3	9		7			
	1		6			7		

Puzzle #24 - Hard

	5		1		8			
8					9			6
7						4		
	6					7	2	
9				3	7	8		5
		7	5	6				
6					5			4
1				4				
		3					9	2

Puzzle #25 - Hard

					1			7
1			7			2	8	
		5			6	3		
	8	7		9				
6				5				8
5			4		8			
		1		8		9	3	
	2		5				1	
	3							4

Puzzle #26 - Hard

8					1	6		
		1	9				4	
			3				8	9
7			8			2		
4		3		5	9			
	8				7		1	
	4					8		1
9					8		5	
	3			6		4		

Puzzle #27 - Hard

					6		2	
6		8	3	1				
	3	4				7		1
		7			1	8		6
	6			3	5			
		3		6				
		6						3
		1	2	9			5	
5							8	9

Puzzle #28 - Hard

9						7	8	
5				8				6
	8	4						5
	6				3	5		
	1			7				
		7	8		2			1
		5	1				2	
8			3		9	1		
				4			3	

Puzzle #29 - Hard

			2		4	7		
					9	1	2	6
			8					
8			9		3			
7		4			1			
		1	5					3
		8						
1						4	7	5
2		7					6	

Puzzle #30 - Hard

			9	6		3	4	
			7		1		2	9
6				7				5
2							8	1
8	5							4
	8	3		1	2			
1	4		3		8			

Puzzle #31 - Hard

9			2	6				
1					7	8		
	5	8						9
					9	2		3
		9	7				1	
				3	4			5
	9					4	3	
	7			8				2
8		6			2			

Puzzle #32 - Hard

4						7		
		5	6				8	
		2	1		9			6
2					4			5
6			7				4	3
		7		2				
					7		1	
				5		4		8
			2	3		5		

Puzzle #33 - Hard

1				8		9		
2							8	
		6	5	4				
7					8			
	9					3		2
3				1		5		
	1		4		7			
		7					1	9
5				9	3	7	6	

Puzzle #34 - Hard

	6		5	3				
		3		6				
		7	1				6	8
		6					3	
5						8	9	
		1		9	2	5		
			6			2		
6		8		1	3			
	3	4					1	7

Puzzle #35 - Hard

				3	2		9	
	8		7					4
					8	1	3	
		7		5			1	
		8				2		3
5	6				1			
8			1	6				
	5	9					8	
4					7	5		

Puzzle #36 - Hard

4		3	6		9			
2	9			1	7			
			1	2		8	3	
				8	3	4		1
	5		7					6
8	1							2
	4					5		8

Puzzle #37 - Hard

					3		6	
			8		9			5
2	9		5				1	
	3	5				6		
		1		8	6		7	
	6						3	
				7	1	3	4	
3	1						8	6
		6	2					

Puzzle #38 - Hard

				8	2			1
7					1		6	
				3			9	7
							3	
		8					4	2
5	4	1						9
					3			
	5			4	8			
6	8	2		1				

Puzzle #39 - Hard

		5	6					3
		4	1		7			
	6	7	2					
	2	1				7	8	
8	7					4		1
				8	2		9	5
			9		4	1	3	

Puzzle #40 - Hard

1		3				9	4	
	5	9					2	8
4	1		8		7			
7		8		1	2			
				7	6	2		
				4		1	7	
	3			5		6		

Puzzle #41 - Hard

	9	3					8	
		1				4	7	
	5			3		1		
			7	5	4		1	
			6			7	2	
						8		
		9	2	6	1			
	2	4			7			
	8							

Puzzle #42 - Hard

	6						7	2
		9	3		7	5	8	
7			6	5				
		8			9	6		
		7					4	
	5			1	8			
		1	4					
3						2		9
		6			5	4		

Puzzle #43 - Hard

		8						
4		2	7					
9			1	2	6			
						8		
				6		7		2
			4	7	5			1
1						4		7
3		9						8
		5			3	1		

Puzzle #44 - Hard

		7	9			3	5	
9						2		
1		6			8			
		5	1		2		3	7
	1					9		
7				6				
		9	8	4			1	
	4			5				
	7	3						8

Puzzle #45 - Hard

				6	9		4	3
			1		7	9	2	
5	8					4		
	2					1	8	
	6			7		5		
8		3	2	1				
4	1		8		3			

Puzzle #46 - Hard

				8			9	
	9	1		2	6	8		5
7					9			
				5				6
6		7	3					
4	8			1				9
		4			1	9	8	
			9				7	1
		3			8			

Puzzle #47 - Hard

	8	1	9		6			
9							3	
				8	2	1		5
	3	4			1		7	
			7			4	6	
					9	8		
7		8		9				
		9			8			
1					5	9		6

Puzzle #48 - Hard

			6		2	4		
				7			5	2
5	4					7		
	8		3		5			6
		1	4				8	
2			7				6	1
		7			4			9
3	5			2				

Puzzle #49 - Hard

			5	9		2		8
				3	1	4	9	
2		1		8	7			
7	8		1		4			
6		7					2	
		4				7	1	
		5	3				6	

Puzzle #50 - Hard

1			7					
	8	4		5				
		5		3	2			
	6		9		1			2
		7				4		
8					6			5
				2				7
4	3				7	6		
	5		4			2		

Puzzle #51 - Hard

				9		7	1	
		3	8					
		4	1			8		9
	7		9					
9		1	6		2		5	8
					8	9		
	6	7		3				
8	4				1		9	
					5		6	

Puzzle #52 - Hard

	8					9	3	
4	7						1	
1			3			5		
					7	2	4	
			6	2	1		9	
						8		
8								
	1		5	7	4			
7	2			6				

Puzzle #53 - Hard

				6		3		
			5	3			6	
6		8	1			7		
3						6		
9	8							5
	5			9	2	1		
	2		6					
1		7				4	3	
				1	3	8		6

Puzzle #54 - Hard

2	3							8
				1		5	6	
		1	5					7
		8					5	9
5				7		4		
			6		1	8		
	4				7		8	
		9	3	2				
1		3		8				

Puzzle #55 - Hard

			3					9
6	9					8	1	
2		8		1	5			
9				8				
	7		6	4				
1			7			3	4	
8							9	
		9					8	7
5				9	6			1

Puzzle #56 - Hard

		3						
	1		2	6	8			
	4	8			5			
			1	5	4	9		
							3	
			8			2	4	
		1		7			6	
	3					7	9	
	8	2				1		

Puzzle #57 - Hard

					7	6		
	9		1					
7		3		5			1	2
				6	1			8
	2				9			
	3	5		7			9	
8			7	3				
			4			5		
		1		9		4	8	

Puzzle #58 - Hard

2				7				
		4			2			5
	7				6	4		3
	1	9		2				6
	6			5		8		
					4		7	
		7				1		
3	2						5	
5							4	8

Puzzle #59 - Hard

		8	7				1	
4	3		9		5			
7				8				2
		4				1		8
9			8				5	
		3			6			4
	1			9			4	
8			1					6
				3		9	8	

Puzzle #60 - Hard

				9			3	2
			1	3				8
		8			4	7		
8			2		3			
	5	6						1
7				1			5	
9		5		8				
	8					1	6	
	4		5					7

Puzzle #61 - Hard

			3		8	2		1
				1	4	8	3	
5				6				7
1	8			2				
4				8	5			
	4	3					9	6
9	2					1	7	

Puzzle #62 - Hard

		5	3			6		
		4				1		7
6		7				2		
2		1		7	8			
7	8		1	4				
				1	3	9		4
			5		9		8	2

Puzzle #63 - Hard

		9		8		5		
3					6			4
4							1	8
			3			8	9	
	1		9			4		
		8		1				6
	3	4		9	5			
8				7		1		
		7	8					2

Puzzle #64 - Hard

		4					8	7
	6		2	4			5	
			9					2
5								6
	8	7		6	1		9	
			3			7		
					4	6	3	
1						5		
8	9			5			7	

Puzzle #65 - Hard

9					5		8	
		4	8	1				
		3	4					6
7			2			8		
4	3						9	5
		8			1		7	
8			6				1	
	1				4	9		
				9	8	3		

Puzzle #66 - Hard

		3	5				1	
		7						8
9			3	2				
		5	7		6		9	3
	7			9	1			
1						4		7
	6					5	4	
		1	9				8	
		2			8			

Puzzle #67 - Hard

8					2			
	9				1		8	
			6				4	5
				1		7		4
1		9	7					
6	7				5	3	9	
					7	8		
	3	2		9				
	5				3		1	

Puzzle #68 - Hard

5				9	3		7	6
		7				9		1
	1		4		7			
7					8			
3				1			5	
	9					2	3	
1				8			9	
2								8
		6	5	4				

Puzzle #69 - Hard

2				6				
			3		1		8	6
	1	7				3	4	
				5	3	6		
					6		3	
	6	8		1			7	
	3						6	
8	9							5
5			2		9		1	

Puzzle #70 - Hard

			1	3			6	8
		2			6			
7	1					3		4
		5	9	2				1
	3							6
	9	8					5	
			6					3
			3		5	6		
8	6				1			7

Puzzle #71 - Hard

		8		6		5		
	6		9	1		2		
7								4
					2	7		
	3	4		7				6
	5		4					2
		1	7					
5				2	3			
4	8				5			

Puzzle #72 - Hard

		8				3	4	
7	4		8					9
	3			1				
					9		1	
2			6			4	8	
		1		4	8			5
	5					6		
8				9	3			
	9	7	1					8

Puzzle #73 - Hard

	3					6		
		6				3		5
	7		8		6			1
				2				6
	4	3	7		1			
6	8					1	3	
	6				3			
	1			5		9	2	
5				8	9			

Puzzle #74 - Hard

		5				1		
	3	6	4					
	7			5		8		9
2					9			
7	8						4	
	5			4	2			6
		7			3			
6						5		
	9		1	6			7	8

Puzzle #75 - Hard

4	5		7					
8				6		5	3	
		1			8		4	
5	3							2
		7		9		4		
	2			1	6		7	
				2	5			7
			4			2	6	

Puzzle #76 - Hard

3	9				8			
	5			1		3		
1				4	7			
	8							
9						6	1	2
4	2						7	
				8				
					1	5	4	7
				7	2			6

Puzzle #77 - Hard

	7							1
3		2				5		
5						4	8	
	4			2			5	
		7		6			3	4
2			7					
	9	1	2				6	
				4		7		
		6	5					8

Puzzle #78 - Hard

		7			9			1
9						2	3	
4	3						5	
2				8	6			
			9			4		3
	8		7				2	
	6	2		9				
7				1		8		
			5		8		9	

Puzzle #79 - Hard

		4	7	1				
6		7		2				
		5		6			3	
7	8						1	4
2		1				8		7
			2		8	9	5	
			4	9		3		1

Puzzle #80 - Hard

		9				5	1	4
	3							
	4	2					8	
	9	7			3			
	6		1			7		
		1	2		8			
			8		4			5
					1	6	2	8
			3					

Puzzle #81 - Hard

3			6	7				
		1	4		8			9
		5						6
	1			4		9	8	
9							7	1
	8			3				
		8					9	
	6	2		1	9	8		5
	9		7					

Puzzle #82 - Hard

	5				8			6
	9					7	8	
4		8						5
		1			7			
		6	3			5		
7			2	8				1
5				1			2	
	8		9	3		1		
					4		3	

Puzzle #83 - Hard

8		4		5				
		1	2	8	6			
3								
		3				7	9	
1					7		6	
2		8				1		
							3	
			1	4	5	9		
			8			2	4	

Puzzle #84 - Hard

8				2		4		
		9	5	3				2
					1	3		
	2				7			
	6		3					8
7			4	9			2	
		5				9		7
1	9						8	
		8			9		6	

Puzzle #85 - Hard

			8	7				9
9	6			1		5		
			9			8		
1	5					2		8
		3		9				
			1		8	6	9	
4		6					7	
		7	4		3	1		
8						9		

Puzzle #86 - Hard

		6		9		8		
		8					1	9
9	7					5		
		2	4		9		7	
	8		3					6
				7				2
	2		5		3	9		
3				1				
4					2		8	

Puzzle #87 - Hard

	3	4		6		7		
					7		2	
	5			2				4
		1						7
5						2	3	
4	8						5	
7				4				
	6				2	1		9
		8			5	6		

Puzzle #88 - Hard

	7	8		1	2			
1	4		8		7			
				4			7	1
				7	6			2
3				5				6
	1	3					4	9
5		9				8	2	

Puzzle #89 - Hard

		7				4		
6			1	9			2	
	8		6				5	
					2		7	
3	4		7			6		
5				4		2		
8		4			5			
	1			7				
		5	2		3			

Puzzle #90 - Hard

	5				6	3		
					1			7
		1		7		2	8	
		6	5					8
8	7		9					
		5		4	8			
	1		8			9	3	
2				5			1	
3								4

Puzzle #91 - Hard

			8		3	4		1
			2	1		8	3	
4						5		8
5				7				6
1	8							2
9	2		1		7			
	4	3		6	9			

Puzzle #92 - Hard

		5	4	8				
8	7				9			
		6			5	8		
		1	7				2	8
	5			6			3	
				1		7		
3						4		
2			5					1
	1				8		9	3

Puzzle #93 - Hard

		2			8			7
			2			6	8	
4	3							9
	1			7		9		
		5	4		3			
2		3	9					
		9				8		5
				2	6		9	
8			7				1	

Puzzle #94 - Hard

				4		6		3
9		8	5					7
		1				5		
		5					6	
					3	7		
8	7		6	1				9
					9		2	
6			4		2			5
	4						7	8

Puzzle #95 - Hard

4		3		5				
9				3	2			
	7		1				9	
2						8	6	
		8		2				7
			3		4			9
7					8	1		
				9			8	5
	2	6				9		

Puzzle #96 - Hard

		7	1					
2	8				7	1		
3			6				5	
	1				5			2
		4						3
9	3			8			1	
				9			7	8
		8		5		6		
			8		4	5		

Puzzle #97 - Hard

					4			5
8				3	7			
	1			9			8	4
			1	6		8		
	5	3		7			9	
		2	9					
7	3			5		2	1	
		9			1			
			7					6

Puzzle #98 - Hard

			8	2			1	
7				1		6		
			3			9	7	
		5	4	8				
				3				
6	2	8	1					
5	1	4					9	
						3		
	8					4	2	

Puzzle #99 - Hard

				1				9
1		2	5			7	3	
	6				7			
		8	6		1			
9			7				5	3
					9			2
8	4		9				1	
			3	7		8		
	5			4				

Puzzle #100 - Hard

1		6	8					
		7		9			3	5
9							2	
	1						9	
		5	2	1		7		3
7					6			
		9		8	4			1
	7	3				8		
	4				5			

Puzzle #101 - Hard

					2		8	1
			5		8			4
		7			6			5
3	8		4		1			
	2	1	8	3				
7	1						2	9
9		6				3	4	

Puzzle #102 - Hard

		5	7		9			
9	1			8				
		8		6				9
	8				4	2		
					3			1
		9	2			3	5	
2								7
6			8				3	
	7			2		9	4	

EXPERT

Puzzle #1 - Expert

						6		
		6	5	4	2	9		
		5	9		6			
					4			
	6				7	3	1	2
	1					4		8
			2					3
5		9		8				
6	7						8	

Puzzle #2 - Expert

	1		9	6		5		
8	7						9	
9						8		
1		8				6		9
			1	5		2	8	
	9				3			
			4		6			7
4		3			7	1		
			8			9		

Puzzle #3 - Expert

	8					9	3	
		1		3		5		
	7	4					1	
		8						
	1		7	5	4			
	2	7	6					
			2	6	1		9	
					7	2	4	
						8		

Puzzle #4 - Expert

	2					6		7
7	1							4
	6			3				5
				1	4	7	8	
			8		7	2		1
4	9		3		1			
2		8	9	5				

Puzzle #5 - Expert

	3	2					8	
				1		6		5
1			5				7	
3		1		8				
9			3	2				
	4				7	8		
8						5	9	
		5		7				4
			6		1			8

Puzzle #6 - Expert

2					7			
		4				8		
1						2	5	3
9	2						6	
	5				9			
			1		3	7		
				4			2	
			2			9	1	8
	9		6					

Puzzle #7 - Expert

2						4		
					9		6	
1	8	9					2	
5	3	2		1				
				2				7
		8	4					
					5			9
		7					1	3
6				9	2			

Puzzle #8 - Expert

							4	
7			3		9			
			1			6		2
	5			6			2	1
	2	8	7					9
	3							8
		4						
2	1			9				
				2	5	9		

Puzzle #9 - Expert

6	9			3	4			
				1			8	
				2	8			3
						5	6	
				6	1		7	
	6	5				9		
	5	9						2
	4					8		
	2	6	4	7				

Puzzle #10 - Expert

2				4				
1	8	9			2			
					6	9		
6						2		9
			9			5		
		7	3		1			
		8					4	
			7					2
5	3	2						1

Puzzle #11 - Expert

			1	9	8	2		
			2				4	
	9					6		
				7		1		3
9	2		6					
	5							9
		4		8				
1			5	2	3			
2								7

Puzzle #12 - Expert

	9		2					
5							4	
			4	5			9	8
	7	5	8					
1				2		6		7
		4			1			
	2			6	3			4
		1				3		
9		3					7	

Puzzle #13 - Expert

	4	2	5					9
	7		6	9			4	
		7		8	3	5		6
	3			5				
		4				9		
				1		6		
		5	7					
7		3		6		1	2	

Puzzle #14 - Expert

	9		4		2	5		
		4	7			6		9
6								1
					5	7		
1		2		7	3			6
9					4			
5	6				7		3	8
			3					5

Puzzle #15 - Expert

8					5			2
		9					8	4
	7				1			
5				1				
			3			4		6
3					4			9
	4	2	1	7				
		3			8		6	
7			6			2		

Puzzle #16 - Expert

2	5			3			7	
				7		4		
	1	6						3
3	2				6			
	7	5	4			8		
				9		2		
		2					1	8
9			2		5			
	3							

Puzzle #17 - Expert

	4			1				
				5		7	4	3
			6					5
	9				4			
				3	2		8	
4	5							1
5					8			
3						2	5	9
		6					7	

Puzzle #18 - Expert

	9				2	6		
		6		5				1
2							7	
	3		7				8	
1	8			2				
7			3	8				
3					5	4		
				9			3	
		9	1					8

Puzzle #19 - Expert

					7	5		9
				3		2		1
					8		3	
5	9		4					8
	6							3
	8		5			4		6
		7		2				
3	1			4				
8	5				6			

Puzzle #20 - Expert

	5	6	2	7				
4					9			
7					8			
	3		5				4	
	6	4				7		
		1				8	3	
			8				9	1
		2		9			8	
			1	4				5

Puzzle #21 - Expert

		4	1					
			5			7	3	4
					6		5	
			3	2				8
	4	5					1	
		9		4				
	3					2	9	5
	5			8				
6								7

Puzzle #22 - Expert

	5		4		2			9
	6	9	7				4	
		6		7	3	1	2	
		1				6		
	7				5			
3		8			7	5		6
					4	9		
		5	3					

Puzzle #23 - Expert

	8				5	4		6
5	9				4			8
	6							3
				7		5		9
				8			3	
			3			2		1
8	5			6				
3	1		4					
		7	2					

Puzzle #24 - Expert

9								4
8								7
	2	7				6	5	
	5				4		3	
			7			4	6	
			8		3	1		
		9			8	2		
	1	4		5				
	8			1	9			

Puzzle #25 - Expert

3		2				9		
		4					7	
	7			5	3			8
6						8		
			6		9	4		2
	2		4					
	6	1	3					
		7		1				
8					4		1	5

Puzzle #26 - Expert

						9		8
	9	4					7	
8		1		5			2	
9	8		3	4				
1		5						
			8		7			
						4		7
				3	6		5	
	2		1		4		6	

Puzzle #27 - Expert

	2				7			
	1					5	3	2
		4						8
				1	3			7
2	9					6		
5					9			
9				6				
				2		1	8	9
			4			2		

Puzzle #28 - Expert

	5		4					
		9					2	
			9		8	5	4	
1				3				
		2			4	6		3
3	9		7					
5		7					8	
	1			6	7	2		
4								1

Puzzle #29 - Expert

1				8			9	
	6		5	4				
2								8
		1	4		7			
5				9	3		7	6
	7					9		1
7					8			
3				1			5	
		9				2	3	

Puzzle #30 - Expert

		7				4	6	
	4				5		3	
	3	8				1		
			8					7
				7	2	6	5	
			9					4
1	9				8			
	8			9		2		
5				4	1			

Puzzle #31 - Expert

				5				9
7						1		3
		6		2	9			
				9		6		
9	8	1				2		
		2					4	
8			4					
					2			7
2	3	5			1			

Puzzle #32 - Expert

9	1		8	6	3			
		3						
5	2			4				
								7
			9	8	6	1	5	
			5			3	8	
			4	5				
7		8					6	
	3					4		2

Puzzle #33 - Expert

					8		6	
	6	9	2		4			
	4					2		
5		3	8			7		
					9		3	2
				7				4
1								7
	3					6		1
		4	5	1			8	

Puzzle #34 - Expert

	1		8		3			
	4	6	7					
		3			4			5
				5		4		1
	2				8	9		
				1	9			8
4							9	
7							8	
	6	5				7		2

Puzzle #35 - Expert

		8		6	4		5	
5		9		8			4	
		6		3				
				1	2			3
			3			8		
				9	5	7		
8		5				6		
3		1						4
	7							2

Puzzle #36 - Expert

	8		7				3	
			3	8		7		
				2		1	8	
	3			9				
8			1					9
		4			5	3		
	7					2		
		6			2		9	
1				5				6

Puzzle #37 - Expert

		4		9	5			
					4	5	3	
								6
3	5				1		9	
7							2	
4			8				5	7
			2	4		8		
	6							
5		1	3					

Puzzle #38 - Expert

		8	5		7			
2				1		7		6
	1		4					
				5			4	
		2			9			
5		4				8	9	
			1					3
			3	9			7	
6	3				2	4		

Puzzle #39 - Expert

				9	1	8	6	3
				5	2		4	
			3					
8	3					5		
		7						
5	1					9	8	6
						4	5	
6			8	7				
	4	2			3			

Puzzle #40 - Expert

3	2				9			
	4		7					
		7		8		3	5	
6					8			
				2	4	9		6
		2						4
	7						1	
8			1	5		4		
	1	6						3

Puzzle #41 - Expert

			5		7			8
			4			1		
6		7		1			2	
		4			2	3	6	
3			1					
	7		3	9				
	4			5				
	9	8					5	4
					9			2

Puzzle #42 - Expert

9								4
			8			3		2
5	4			1				
	5							8
	3		5	9	2			
		6	7					
4						1		
			4	3	7	5		
				5			6	

Puzzle #43 - Expert

		7					6	5
6	1			5	8		9	
					3			
2							4	
					6			9
1	6		9		5			
7								
3		5	4		7			2
				3			7	4

Puzzle #44 - Expert

		2					7	
		4				3		1
	6					8		5
		3	1		2			
	8			3				
	7		9		5			
			3					6
4			8			5		9
5			6		4			8

Puzzle #45 - Expert

		4		8			5	1
	3		6		1			
1					7			
					4			7
5		3	7				8	
				3	2	9		
	4		2					
	6	9				4	2	
				6		8		

Puzzle #46 - Expert

	3		7					
					6		5	
1		6		9		8		7
		5		7		9	8	
4			6	3				
			5				1	
				8	7			4
	9				2			
	2	4		5		6		

Puzzle #47 - Expert

	2			3			1	7
9						3	8	
		6			9			
		5	9				2	8
2				5				
					1	7		3
6				4				
	7		3			8		
		1			8			

Puzzle #48 - Expert

9	3							7
		2		3	6		4	
	1					3		
	5	7	8					
1					2	6	7	
	4			1				
		9	2					
			4		5		8	9
5								4

Puzzle #49 - Expert

				9			5	6
			6	5				
1		6	7					
	4	7					6	2
				8				4
					2		9	5
8		2			3			
		1	8					
4		3				6		9

Puzzle #50 - Expert

	7				4		8	
	6		3					
				7		4	9	
		8					4	2
1					3			
	2				6		5	
4		5	1	3				
	1			9		5		
		7			2			9

Puzzle #51 - Expert

								4
	9					2	1	
	2	5			9			
				8			3	
	6		2	1			5	
7				9			2	8
			4					
3		9				7		
1				2	6			

Puzzle #52 - Expert

		4					2	
9			3		7			
	6						5	
				3				8
			7					1
2		8			4			
	3		2				9	
		5		6				2
	2	7	5	1		3		

Puzzle #53 - Expert

	5	4						
					3	4	2	
			7	8				6
							7	
		5				3		8
6	8	9				1		5
3	6	8	9		1			
	4		5		2			
				3				

Puzzle #54 - Expert

9						7		3
		6			5			
	4				2			
	5		2				6	
	7	2		3			1	5
		3			9			2
			8				3	
			1					7
2	8					4		

EXTREME

Puzzle #1 - Extreme

	6				8			
	8	7		4				
3		5	2					
	1							7
9		3				6		
6	5						9	
			8	6		3	7	
		6			1		5	9
1				5	7			2

Puzzle #2 - Extreme

	8		4			5		
		1		8				
4			5		3			
			7				9	
				2	6			5
	9			3		7		
2				9		4	1	
	6	4	1					9
		8			5		7	

Puzzle #3 - Extreme

			8		2			1
5		6				9		
7	8			1	5		6	
			5					8
8				2			3	7
	4				8		1	
		3				8		
1				8			7	
	9				7	1	2	

Puzzle #4 - Extreme

					1	9	5	
					3		4	6
			7	6				2
6		7			9	8		
	1			7			6	9
	3		5			2		
1		2		3				
3			1		2			
	8	9		4				

Puzzle #5 - Extreme

3		4		6				
	7	1			2	5		
6	8							
				5	9			
		5	4		3			6
	9		1	8		3		
					7	8	2	
		8		9		1		3
							9	7

Puzzle #6 - Extreme

				7				9
		9			3	7		
			6		2		5	
		8		4		5		
	4		3	5				
1					8			
	2				9	4		1
8			5					7
4		6		1			9	

Puzzle #7 - Extreme

								9
		4			5	6	3	
	2		7			4	8	
								6
		3			6	8	1	
	7		1			2	9	
9				6				
	6	1	5		8			
	4	7	9		2			

Puzzle #8 - Extreme

			4				8	7
				8			6	
					2	3		5
		6				9		3
	7						1	
9						6	5	
5	9			1				6
	2		5	7		1		
7		3	6		8			

Puzzle #9 - Extreme

5							2	6
		7			9		3	
	9					7		
			1				8	
		5			8	4		
				4		5		3
9			4		6	1		
	7		8					5
	1	4		2			9	

Puzzle #10 - Extreme

	8	7						4
	6					8		
3		5					2	
				3	7		8	6
1			2			7		5
		6	9		5	1		
6	5				9			
	1		7					
9		3		6				

Puzzle #11 - Extreme

	2		8		3		4	
	8			6			5	
	1			2			9	
9								5
1	6			4		8		
		3						4
2								9
		6		9			2	7
8						1		

Puzzle #12 - Extreme

9		6			1		7	
	2				3	5		
	8		6	7				9
6		4						3
2						7	6	
	9	5						1
				9	8		4	
			3			1		2
			1	2			3	

Puzzle #13 - Extreme

		9				6	2	
		6				4		5
8	2							9
		7	3		4		6	
9				2		3		1
	5			1			7	
6			1	3				
	3	1			8			
7			2		9			

Puzzle #14 - Extreme

8				6		5		
1				2		9		
2			3		8	4		
	3							4
6		1		4			8	
		9						5
		2						9
		8					1	
	6			9		2		7

Puzzle #15 - Extreme

		1				8		
	8		5					4
4							3	5
				9				7
	9		7			3		
					5	2	6	
2			4	1		9		
	6	4			9			1
		8		7			5	

Puzzle #16 - Extreme

7		9		1			3	
			8					
	2	8						1
	4		2				6	9
9		6			5		4	
	7		6		9			8
								6
3		7			6	4		
6	8		5					

Puzzle #17 - Extreme

1	6						9	5
2					4			
			9					6
								3
		7	5		6			
6	1				9	5		8
			4		7	3		
3		5	2				4	7
7								

Puzzle #18 - Extreme

4	9	5		2				
				7	9		5	4
			1			8		
2	1	8				6		
			8		2	1	9	
				6				3
8								
	2	6		9		4		
3								

Puzzle #19 - Extreme

8	3		7	6		1		
		2				5		7
7				2			3	
	1		2			9		
2	6			3		8	7	
		9		5	8			
			4			7		
				1			9	
					3			4

Puzzle #20 - Extreme

	8				9			6
4							2	
		1				8		4
3				6		5		
		8		2	3		9	
5	4		7					1
			9			7	1	
				5				9
	5				7		4	

Puzzle #21 - Extreme

					3		6	
	4		9			8		
8				1		7	5	
2				8		1		
	8		7			5		2
		5						8
3	1		2	7		6		
			1		8		9	
7		8						1

Puzzle #22 - Extreme

			6		4		3	
4								
	6		9	8		1		
		8	4	7		2		
7					6	8	9	
3		6			9		7	
							1	
		5	2	6				8
6				9	5			

Puzzle #23 - Extreme

	1	9				3	8	
	8	2				6	4	
6								9
	3		1	7		4		
					9			
		7	6	4			2	
		1	5	9			7	
	6		8	2		5		
					6			

Puzzle #24 - Extreme

		6	5				8	
3	8		4				2	
		2	9				1	
		9	2		7	6		
					9			2
				1				8
					4	3		
					5			9
		4		8			6	1

Puzzle #25 - Extreme

2	8				7			
9		7						
	1	3	9					8
			5		9			
	3		8	1			9	
		6		4	3			5
	5				2		7	1
						6	8	
			6			3		4

Puzzle #26 - Extreme

				4				
		1	6				9	8
3						4	6	
1								
	8				5		2	6
				6		5		9
7				3	6	9		
9		8		7		6		
		2			8		4	7

Puzzle #27 - Extreme

		9				6		
7	4						9	2
1	6						5	8
	2		4		8	7		
4			6		3			5
				9				
	7		2		9		1	
3			8		1			6
				6				

Puzzle #28 - Extreme

		9					1	
	4					3		
7								4
					9	8	5	
8		7	2	6			3	
9				1				2
1			8	3			6	7
		3	7				2	
5	7				2			

Puzzle #29 - Extreme

	7				4	6		9
2	4		9			5		
5						7		
				6				1
3		7		1	2			6
4				9				
	3							5
7			6	5			3	8

Puzzle #30 - Extreme

		5			8	4		
			4			5		3
				1			8	
5							2	6
		7			9		3	
	9					7		
	7			8				5
9				4	6	1		
	1	4	2				9	

Puzzle #31 - Extreme

			5		6	7		
	5	8			9		6	1
		3						
							7	
	3		4	7				
4		7	2			5	3	
9		5					1	6
		6	9					
					4		2	

Puzzle #32 - Extreme

	4			5			8	
8						1		
	5	3						4
3				7			9	
2		6			5			
	7		9					
		5	7			8		
9			1	4				2
	1				9	4	6	

Puzzle #33 - Extreme

	1				7		5	
	2		3	1				9
3		4			6	7		
			4	5		6		
			6		2	9		
				9			2	8
2		9						7
1	3							6
		8				1	3	

Puzzle #34 - Extreme

8	5			1	6			
2	9			7	4			
		6	9					
6				3			8	1
	1				7		2	9
						6		
						9		
	7				2		4	8
5				4			6	3

Puzzle #35 - Extreme

	7		9					
2		6		5				
3					7	9		
9			1		4		2	
		5	7					8
	1			9		6		4
	5	3					4	
8								1
	4				5	8		

Puzzle #36 - Extreme

	3		9		7		1	
						8		
1			8	2				
		4	7		3			6
				8	6	5		
6								
	4		6		9			5
8				7		6		9
9	6			4		2		

Puzzle #37 - Extreme

	8	9		1			6	
4		6			3			
						4		
6				8	9	7		
9					7	3		6
	7	4		2				8
	6	2	8					5
					1			
5	9					6		

Puzzle #38 - Extreme

		4					9	
	3			5				
		7		8	3		5	6
	4	2	5					9
	7		6	9		4		
		5	7					
				1			6	
7		3		6		2	1	

Puzzle #39 - Extreme

						5		9
3			9			8	1	
	6			5			4	3
1	3			8		9		
	7	9						
8		2						7
5			7	1				2
				4	3	6		
			8		6			

Puzzle #40 - Extreme

	2	8	9	1				
6					3			
				6		2	8	1
7	9		5		4			
2						4	5	9
		1		8				
						8		
						3		
9				4			6	2

Puzzle #41 - Extreme

				7			1	
					9		5	6
			6			3		9
	4					7	8	
8							6	
		2				5		3
7	5			2				1
1				9	5	6		
	6	8	3		7			

Puzzle #42 - Extreme

			4					3
				9		1		
					7		4	
3	8				1	6	7	
	7			3		2		
		2	7		5			
1					9		2	
		9				5		8
6	2			7	8	3		

Puzzle #43 - Extreme

					5	8		
		7		8		2	5	
8			2				1	
	3							6
		9		4			8	
1			8				7	5
7		2	3	1			6	
			7		8	1		
	8	1						9

Puzzle #44 - Extreme

			8	7		2		
			3			6	1	
					2			9
4			7				2	
	3							8
		1	6	2		3		5
7			1		5	8	9	
		9		3		7		
	4				7			

Puzzle #45 - Extreme

			1	2	8	6		
2		8				1	9	
	6							3
				3				
	9		2		6	4		
				8				
9	7						5	4
	2		9	4	5			
		1				8		

Puzzle #46 - Extreme

6	1			5	8			
4	7			9	2			
		9	6					
	4				5		3	6
						9		
2				7			8	4
	3				6		1	8
						6		
7				1			9	2

Puzzle #47 - Extreme

				9				
4			1		7	3		
	2		6		4		7	
3	8					1	9	
		9						6
6	4					8	2	
5			8		2	6		
	7		5		9		1	
				6				

Puzzle #48 - Extreme

4					9	6		2
							8	
							3	
6						8	2	1
	3				6			
1		9	8	2				
					2	5	4	9
	4	5		9	7			
8			1					

Puzzle #49 - Extreme

7					9	1	2	
			3			8		
		8		1			7	
2	8							1
5		1		7	8		6	
			6	5		9		
8					4		1	
		2		8			3	7
	5							8

Puzzle #50 - Extreme

	1			9		6	4	
		9	1		4			2
5			7				8	
3	5							4
		8					1	
	4				5	8		
	7		9					
6		2		5				
		3			7	9		

Puzzle #51 - Extreme

		6		1			9	5
			8		6	3		7
	1			7	5		2	
5	6							9
	9	3				6		
1							7	
6				8				
	3	5	2					
8		7			4			

Puzzle #52 - Extreme

	7	8			9			
3		6						
4	1		5			8		
6				5	8	9		
			4		1			
	2		3	9			7	
			6			3		7
	5				3	1	8	
							2	9

Puzzle #53 - Extreme

		8		3	7	2		
	4			1				8
					8		5	
					1		8	2
	8	7		6		1		5
6		5	9					
		1		7		8		
3			8					
	9		1	2				7

Puzzle #54 - Extreme

	5	9	1	6				
	6						9	
			2					4
			7					
	7	4	3		5		2	
3							4	7
	3							
					7		5	6
5	8		6	1				9

ANSWERS

Puzzle #1 - Easy

4	7	2	3	8	6	9	1	5
9	3	1	2	5	7	6	4	8
5	8	6	4	9	1	2	3	7
7	4	5	9	3	8	1	6	2
3	2	9	6	1	5	8	7	4
1	6	8	7	2	4	3	5	9
8	1	7	5	6	9	4	2	3
6	5	3	8	4	2	7	9	1
2	9	4	1	7	3	5	8	6

Puzzle #2 - Easy

7	4	5	8	3	2	6	9	1
3	2	9	4	6	1	5	7	8
6	1	8	7	9	5	3	4	2
2	8	6	3	7	4	9	1	5
1	7	3	2	5	9	8	6	4
9	5	4	1	8	6	7	2	3
8	9	1	6	4	3	2	5	7
4	6	7	5	2	8	1	3	9
5	3	2	9	1	7	4	8	6

Puzzle #3 - Easy

2	3	8	7	1	9	6	5	4
7	6	4	5	3	8	2	9	1
1	5	9	4	2	6	3	8	7
3	9	2	6	8	4	7	1	5
6	4	1	2	7	5	9	3	8
5	8	7	1	9	3	4	2	6
4	2	6	3	5	1	8	7	9
8	7	5	9	6	2	1	4	3
9	1	3	8	4	7	5	6	2

Puzzle #4 - Easy

2	4	9	3	1	6	7	5	8
1	8	3	4	7	5	2	9	6
6	7	5	2	9	8	3	1	4
8	5	4	9	2	3	1	6	7
9	6	7	5	8	1	4	3	2
3	1	2	6	4	7	9	8	5
5	9	8	7	3	4	6	2	1
7	3	1	8	6	2	5	4	9
4	2	6	1	5	9	8	7	3

Puzzle #5 - Easy

1	7	3	9	8	2	5	6	4
4	6	9	3	7	5	8	2	1
2	8	5	4	6	1	3	7	9
8	3	6	2	4	7	9	1	5
7	2	4	5	1	9	6	3	8
9	5	1	6	3	8	2	4	7
6	9	2	7	5	4	1	8	3
5	1	7	8	2	3	4	9	6
3	4	8	1	9	6	7	5	2

Puzzle #6 - Easy

9	6	2	1	3	4	5	7	8
4	1	8	9	7	5	2	3	6
3	7	5	6	2	8	9	1	4
7	5	1	3	8	9	4	6	2
2	3	9	4	6	7	8	5	1
8	4	6	5	1	2	3	9	7
1	8	4	7	5	3	6	2	9
6	2	3	8	9	1	7	4	5
5	9	7	2	4	6	1	8	3

Puzzle #7 - Easy

4	9	7	6	3	2	1	5	8
8	6	1	9	4	5	2	3	7
2	3	5	8	1	7	4	6	9
9	7	3	1	2	4	6	8	5
6	2	4	5	9	8	3	7	1
5	1	8	3	7	6	9	2	4
3	4	6	7	5	1	8	9	2
1	5	9	2	8	3	7	4	6
7	8	2	4	6	9	5	1	3

Puzzle #8 - Easy

2	7	3	5	4	6	9	1	8
1	6	5	3	9	8	7	4	2
8	4	9	2	1	7	5	3	6
5	3	2	8	7	9	4	6	1
6	9	4	1	5	3	2	8	7
7	1	8	6	2	4	3	9	5
3	2	1	9	6	5	8	7	4
9	5	7	4	8	1	6	2	3
4	8	6	7	3	2	1	5	9

Puzzle #9 - Easy

7	9	3	2	4	5	8	6	1
8	1	5	6	3	7	4	9	2
4	6	2	9	1	8	7	5	3
2	7	8	5	9	4	3	1	6
3	5	6	7	2	1	9	8	4
1	4	9	3	8	6	2	7	5
9	8	4	1	6	3	5	2	7
6	3	7	8	5	2	1	4	9
5	2	1	4	7	9	6	3	8

Puzzle #10 - Easy

6	4	2	1	9	5	3	8	7
9	7	1	2	8	3	6	5	4
8	5	3	7	4	6	2	9	1
7	8	4	9	3	1	5	6	2
2	9	6	8	5	7	1	4	3
1	3	5	4	6	2	8	7	9
3	1	9	5	7	8	4	2	6
4	6	8	3	2	9	7	1	5
5	2	7	6	1	4	9	3	8

Puzzle #11 - Easy

6	1	4	7	8	2	9	5	3
8	9	7	5	3	6	4	2	1
3	5	2	1	4	9	6	8	7
1	4	3	9	5	8	2	7	6
5	7	8	6	2	3	1	9	4
9	2	6	4	7	1	8	3	5
7	8	9	3	6	4	5	1	2
4	3	1	2	9	5	7	6	8
2	6	5	8	1	7	3	4	9

Puzzle #12 - Easy

7	8	2	4	9	1	3	5	6
1	5	4	6	2	3	7	8	9
3	6	9	7	8	5	2	1	4
9	2	7	8	5	6	4	3	1
5	1	3	2	7	4	9	6	8
8	4	6	3	1	9	5	2	7
2	7	1	5	4	8	6	9	3
4	3	8	9	6	2	1	7	5
6	9	5	1	3	7	8	4	2

Puzzle #13 - Easy

6	3	2	5	4	1	9	8	7
4	1	9	8	2	7	6	5	3
7	5	8	6	9	3	4	1	2
3	9	1	4	6	8	7	2	5
2	4	7	1	3	5	8	6	9
8	6	5	2	7	9	1	3	4
1	7	3	9	5	6	2	4	8
5	8	4	7	1	2	3	9	6
9	2	6	3	8	4	5	7	1

Puzzle #14 - Easy

5	3	1	4	9	6	8	7	2
7	6	4	2	3	8	5	1	9
8	2	9	7	1	5	4	3	6
1	8	5	6	2	3	9	4	7
2	7	3	9	5	4	6	8	1
4	9	6	8	7	1	3	2	5
3	1	7	5	8	9	2	6	4
9	4	2	3	6	7	1	5	8
6	5	8	1	4	2	7	9	3

Puzzle #15 - Easy

3	9	4	5	6	1	2	7	8
7	6	1	9	2	8	3	5	4
5	2	8	7	3	4	9	1	6
2	3	7	4	9	5	6	8	1
6	1	9	2	8	7	4	3	5
8	4	5	6	1	3	7	9	2
9	5	2	1	7	6	8	4	3
4	8	6	3	5	9	1	2	7
1	7	3	8	4	2	5	6	9

Puzzle #16 - Easy

4	5	7	3	6	2	8	9	1
2	9	6	4	1	8	7	5	3
8	3	1	7	5	9	2	4	6
1	4	9	5	3	7	6	2	8
7	8	5	2	9	6	1	3	4
3	6	2	8	4	1	9	7	5
6	2	4	1	7	5	3	8	9
9	7	3	6	8	4	5	1	2
5	1	8	9	2	3	4	6	7

Puzzle #17 - Easy

9	4	6	3	2	8	5	7	1
8	1	3	4	5	7	6	2	9
5	7	2	6	9	1	3	8	4
6	5	4	2	8	9	1	3	7
7	3	9	1	6	4	2	5	8
2	8	1	5	7	3	4	9	6
4	2	7	8	3	6	9	1	5
3	6	8	9	1	5	7	4	2
1	9	5	7	4	2	8	6	3

Puzzle #18 - Easy

8	1	9	3	7	5	6	4	2
2	4	3	1	8	6	7	5	9
6	7	5	9	2	4	3	8	1
3	5	2	6	1	8	9	7	4
4	8	7	2	3	9	5	1	6
9	6	1	4	5	7	8	2	3
5	2	4	7	6	3	1	9	8
1	3	8	5	9	2	4	6	7
7	9	6	8	4	1	2	3	5

Puzzle #19 - Easy

9	7	5	1	2	6	3	4	8
8	6	4	7	5	3	1	2	9
1	2	3	9	8	4	7	6	5
6	8	9	2	1	7	4	5	3
4	5	1	6	3	8	2	9	7
7	3	2	4	9	5	8	1	6
2	1	6	3	7	9	5	8	4
5	4	7	8	6	2	9	3	1
3	9	8	5	4	1	6	7	2

Puzzle #20 - Easy

2	3	7	1	6	8	9	5	4
6	1	9	5	4	3	8	7	2
8	4	5	2	7	9	1	3	6
5	2	8	6	9	1	3	4	7
7	6	1	4	3	5	2	8	9
3	9	4	8	2	7	6	1	5
1	7	3	9	5	6	4	2	8
4	8	6	7	1	2	5	9	3
9	5	2	3	8	4	7	6	1

Puzzle #21 - Easy

1	6	7	8	2	4	9	5	3
3	4	9	7	5	6	8	1	2
2	8	5	1	3	9	4	6	7
6	3	8	2	7	5	1	9	4
5	2	1	4	9	3	7	8	6
9	7	4	6	8	1	2	3	5
4	9	3	5	1	7	6	2	8
8	1	6	3	4	2	5	7	9
7	5	2	9	6	8	3	4	1

Puzzle #22 - Easy

8	2	5	3	7	4	6	9	1
1	6	7	2	9	8	4	3	5
4	9	3	6	5	1	8	2	7
5	4	8	1	6	3	2	7	9
9	1	6	8	2	7	5	4	3
7	3	2	9	4	5	1	6	8
6	8	4	5	3	9	7	1	2
3	7	1	4	8	2	9	5	6
2	5	9	7	1	6	3	8	4

Puzzle #23 - Easy

3	9	1	6	8	4	5	7	2
8	6	5	7	9	2	4	1	3
2	4	7	3	5	1	9	8	6
4	1	9	2	7	8	3	6	5
7	5	8	9	3	6	2	4	1
6	3	2	4	1	5	7	9	8
1	7	3	5	6	9	8	2	4
9	2	6	8	4	3	1	5	7
5	8	4	1	2	7	6	3	9

Puzzle #24- Easy

2	1	7	8	9	6	3	4	5
9	3	8	5	7	4	1	6	2
6	5	4	3	1	2	9	8	7
1	8	5	2	6	3	4	7	9
4	7	6	9	5	8	2	1	3
3	9	2	1	4	7	6	5	8
5	6	3	4	8	9	7	2	1
8	4	9	7	2	1	5	3	6
7	2	1	6	3	5	8	9	4

Puzzle #25 - Easy

1	4	3	6	5	7	9	2	8
9	6	2	1	3	8	7	4	5
5	8	7	2	9	4	1	3	6
4	9	5	7	1	3	6	8	2
2	1	6	5	8	9	3	7	4
7	3	8	4	6	2	5	1	9
3	2	4	9	7	6	8	5	1
8	5	9	3	2	1	4	6	7
6	7	1	8	4	5	2	9	3

Puzzle #26 - Easy

9	8	7	1	4	2	6	5	3
1	6	2	3	8	5	9	7	4
5	4	3	9	6	7	1	8	2
3	2	1	5	9	6	8	4	7
4	9	6	8	7	3	2	1	5
7	5	8	2	1	4	3	6	9
8	7	5	6	3	9	4	2	1
2	1	9	4	5	8	7	3	6
6	3	4	7	2	1	5	9	8

Puzzle #27 - Easy

7	3	2	4	5	9	1	6	8
8	5	1	3	2	6	7	9	4
9	6	4	1	7	8	5	3	2
1	7	3	9	8	5	4	2	6
4	2	9	7	6	3	8	1	5
5	8	6	2	4	1	3	7	9
6	4	7	8	3	2	9	5	1
2	9	8	5	1	7	6	4	3
3	1	5	6	9	4	2	8	7

Puzzle #28 - Easy

8	5	1	6	7	3	9	4	2
3	9	7	4	2	1	6	5	8
4	6	2	8	9	5	3	1	7
2	7	8	9	6	4	5	3	1
6	3	4	1	5	7	8	2	9
9	1	5	3	8	2	7	6	4
5	2	3	7	1	8	4	9	6
7	4	9	2	3	6	1	8	5
1	8	6	5	4	9	2	7	3

Puzzle #29 - Easy

9	2	3	4	6	1	8	5	7
4	8	1	5	3	7	9	2	6
7	5	6	9	8	2	1	4	3
5	6	9	2	1	3	4	7	8
2	3	8	7	4	5	6	9	1
1	7	4	8	9	6	2	3	5
8	9	7	6	5	4	3	1	2
6	1	5	3	2	9	7	8	4
3	4	2	1	7	8	5	6	9

Puzzle #30 - Easy

1	3	7	2	8	4	9	6	5
5	4	8	3	6	9	7	2	1
9	6	2	5	1	7	3	4	8
4	9	1	6	3	5	8	7	2
7	8	5	4	2	1	6	3	9
6	2	3	9	7	8	5	1	4
2	7	4	8	9	6	1	5	3
3	1	9	7	5	2	4	8	6
8	5	6	1	4	3	2	9	7

Puzzle #31 - Easy

5	8	3	7	4	9	2	6	1
7	6	9	8	2	1	3	4	5
2	4	1	5	3	6	7	8	9
3	7	8	1	5	2	6	9	4
6	9	5	4	7	8	1	2	3
4	1	2	6	9	3	8	5	7
1	2	7	9	8	5	4	3	6
8	5	4	3	6	7	9	1	2
9	3	6	2	1	4	5	7	8

Puzzle #32 - Easy

2	5	3	6	8	4	1	7	9
1	8	9	7	5	2	4	3	6
7	4	6	9	3	1	2	8	5
3	1	7	4	6	8	5	9	2
6	2	8	5	1	9	7	4	3
4	9	5	3	2	7	8	6	1
8	6	1	2	4	3	9	5	7
5	7	4	1	9	6	3	2	8
9	3	2	8	7	5	6	1	4

Puzzle #33 - Easy

4	6	8	7	1	2	5	3	9
1	3	7	9	5	6	4	8	2
9	2	5	3	8	4	7	1	6
3	4	9	8	2	7	6	5	1
5	8	2	6	9	1	3	7	4
7	1	6	4	3	5	2	9	8
8	5	4	2	7	9	1	6	3
6	9	1	5	4	3	8	2	7
2	7	3	1	6	8	9	4	5

Puzzle #34 - Easy

5	7	1	4	6	9	8	2	3
3	8	4	7	2	5	1	9	6
6	2	9	1	3	8	7	5	4
7	4	2	6	8	3	5	1	9
8	6	3	9	5	1	2	4	7
9	1	5	2	7	4	6	3	8
2	5	8	3	9	7	4	6	1
4	9	6	8	1	2	3	7	5
1	3	7	5	4	6	9	8	2

Puzzle #35 - Easy

6	2	9	3	5	7	8	1	4
7	4	5	1	9	8	2	6	3
1	8	3	6	4	2	9	5	7
2	3	6	5	7	9	1	4	8
5	7	8	4	3	1	6	9	2
9	1	4	8	2	6	7	3	5
8	5	1	7	6	4	3	2	9
4	6	2	9	8	3	5	7	1
3	9	7	2	1	5	4	8	6

Puzzle #36 - Easy

6	2	7	3	4	1	9	5	8
5	8	3	6	2	9	4	7	1
4	1	9	8	7	5	6	2	3
1	4	2	7	9	8	5	3	6
3	9	5	4	1	6	7	8	2
7	6	8	2	5	3	1	4	9
8	7	6	1	3	4	2	9	5
2	5	1	9	8	7	3	6	4
9	3	4	5	6	2	8	1	7

Puzzle #37 - Easy

6	4	5	1	3	2	7	8	9
1	9	3	8	7	5	4	6	2
8	2	7	4	6	9	5	1	3
7	3	6	2	1	4	8	9	5
5	8	4	3	9	6	2	7	1
9	1	2	5	8	7	3	4	6
4	7	1	9	2	3	6	5	8
3	5	9	6	4	8	1	2	7
2	6	8	7	5	1	9	3	4

Puzzle #38 - Easy

7	4	2	5	9	1	8	3	6
9	1	5	6	8	3	7	4	2
8	6	3	2	7	4	5	1	9
5	7	1	8	3	2	6	9	4
6	2	9	7	4	5	3	8	1
3	8	4	1	6	9	2	5	7
2	5	8	4	1	6	9	7	3
1	3	7	9	2	8	4	6	5
4	9	6	3	5	7	1	2	8

Puzzle #39 - Easy

6	8	4	2	1	5	9	7	3
1	7	5	9	8	3	6	2	4
9	2	3	7	6	4	5	1	8
4	1	8	3	5	7	2	9	6
7	5	9	6	4	2	8	3	1
3	6	2	1	9	8	4	5	7
2	9	6	4	3	1	7	8	5
8	4	1	5	7	9	3	6	2
5	3	7	8	2	6	1	4	9

Puzzle #40 - Easy

8	7	5	6	4	3	2	9	1
3	1	9	2	8	5	6	7	4
6	2	4	1	9	7	8	3	5
4	6	7	9	1	8	5	2	3
5	8	3	7	2	6	4	1	9
1	9	2	5	3	4	7	6	8
9	5	1	4	6	2	3	8	7
7	3	6	8	5	9	1	4	2
2	4	8	3	7	1	9	5	6

Puzzle #41 - Easy

8	7	5	4	9	1	6	2	3
6	2	9	5	3	8	4	7	1
3	4	1	6	7	2	9	5	8
2	5	3	7	8	6	1	4	9
4	1	6	3	5	9	7	8	2
7	9	8	1	2	4	5	3	6
1	3	4	8	6	7	2	9	5
5	6	2	9	4	3	8	1	7
9	8	7	2	1	5	3	6	4

Puzzle #42 - Easy

4	9	6	1	7	5	8	3	2
7	5	2	4	8	3	1	6	9
1	8	3	9	2	6	7	4	5
9	1	5	3	6	8	2	7	4
6	3	8	2	4	7	5	9	1
2	4	7	5	1	9	6	8	3
5	6	4	7	3	1	9	2	8
3	7	9	8	5	2	4	1	6
8	2	1	6	9	4	3	5	7

Puzzle #43 - Easy

8	4	7	3	2	9	1	5	6
3	9	5	1	6	8	2	4	7
1	2	6	7	4	5	3	8	9
5	6	8	2	9	4	7	3	1
7	1	9	6	5	3	4	2	8
4	3	2	8	1	7	6	9	5
9	5	1	4	7	2	8	6	3
6	8	4	9	3	1	5	7	2
2	7	3	5	8	6	9	1	4

Puzzle #44 - Easy

3	5	4	9	8	2	6	1	7
2	7	8	5	1	6	9	4	3
9	1	6	7	4	3	2	8	5
5	6	9	8	2	4	7	3	1
8	4	3	1	6	7	5	2	9
1	2	7	3	9	5	8	6	4
7	9	2	6	3	1	4	5	8
6	8	1	4	5	9	3	7	2
4	3	5	2	7	8	1	9	6

Puzzle #45 - Easy

1	4	6	9	3	5	2	8	7
5	2	3	6	7	8	9	4	1
9	7	8	4	1	2	6	3	5
3	1	4	7	8	6	5	9	2
6	5	2	3	9	4	7	1	8
8	9	7	5	2	1	4	6	3
2	6	9	8	5	3	1	7	4
7	8	5	1	4	9	3	2	6
4	3	1	2	6	7	8	5	9

Puzzle #46 - Easy

1	9	4	8	5	3	7	2	6
2	3	5	6	4	7	9	1	8
6	8	7	9	1	2	5	3	4
3	5	8	2	6	4	1	9	7
7	4	6	1	3	9	2	8	5
9	1	2	7	8	5	6	4	3
5	6	9	4	2	8	3	7	1
4	2	1	3	7	6	8	5	9
8	7	3	5	9	1	4	6	2

Puzzle #47 - Easy

7	5	8	4	1	2	6	9	3
1	9	2	7	6	3	4	8	5
3	4	6	5	8	9	7	1	2
4	3	5	1	2	8	9	7	6
8	7	9	6	3	5	1	2	4
6	2	1	9	4	7	3	5	8
9	6	4	2	5	1	8	3	7
5	8	7	3	9	6	2	4	1
2	1	3	8	7	4	5	6	9

Puzzle #48 - Easy

2	9	3	8	5	7	1	6	4
8	4	1	9	2	6	7	3	5
5	7	6	1	4	3	2	8	9
7	1	4	2	3	5	6	9	8
6	5	9	4	7	8	3	1	2
3	2	8	6	9	1	5	4	7
4	3	2	5	6	9	8	7	1
9	8	7	3	1	2	4	5	6
1	6	5	7	8	4	9	2	3

Puzzle #49 - Easy

6	9	3	1	7	2	5	8	4
8	4	2	5	9	6	1	7	3
1	7	5	8	3	4	9	2	6
3	5	6	2	8	7	4	1	9
7	8	9	4	5	1	6	3	2
2	1	4	9	6	3	7	5	8
4	3	1	7	2	9	8	6	5
5	2	7	6	4	8	3	9	1
9	6	8	3	1	5	2	4	7

Puzzle #50 - Easy

3	7	1	6	9	5	8	2	4
6	2	9	4	3	8	1	5	7
4	8	5	2	7	1	6	3	9
8	5	7	3	6	9	2	4	1
9	1	4	7	8	2	3	6	5
2	3	6	1	5	4	7	9	8
7	4	2	5	1	3	9	8	6
1	9	3	8	4	6	5	7	2
5	6	8	9	2	7	4	1	3

Puzzle #51 - Easy

1	9	6	5	4	3	7	2	8
3	7	2	1	6	8	5	4	9
4	5	8	2	7	9	3	6	1
5	2	9	3	8	4	6	1	7
8	6	4	7	1	2	9	3	5
7	3	1	9	5	6	2	8	4
2	8	5	6	9	1	4	7	3
6	1	7	4	3	5	8	9	2
9	4	3	8	2	7	1	5	6

Puzzle #52 - Easy

2	4	1	5	3	6	8	7	9
5	9	3	7	8	2	6	4	1
8	6	7	1	4	9	3	2	5
9	1	4	6	2	3	5	8	7
7	2	6	9	5	8	1	3	4
3	8	5	4	7	1	9	6	2
4	3	9	8	1	7	2	5	6
1	5	2	3	6	4	7	9	8
6	7	8	2	9	5	4	1	3

Puzzle #53 - Easy

7	9	8	5	4	1	6	2	3
3	6	5	8	2	7	4	9	1
2	4	1	6	9	3	7	8	5
8	2	4	9	5	6	1	3	7
1	5	7	3	8	4	9	6	2
6	3	9	7	1	2	5	4	8
4	1	3	2	7	9	8	5	6
5	7	2	4	6	8	3	1	9
9	8	6	1	3	5	2	7	4

Puzzle #54- Easy

3	1	4	8	6	7	9	5	2
8	9	7	2	1	5	6	4	3
6	5	2	9	4	3	1	7	8
5	2	3	7	8	6	4	9	1
9	7	8	1	2	4	3	6	5
1	4	6	3	5	9	8	2	7
2	6	9	5	3	8	7	1	4
7	8	5	4	9	1	2	3	6
4	3	1	6	7	2	5	8	9

Puzzle #55 - Easy

6	9	8	1	4	3	7	5	2
1	5	7	8	2	6	4	9	3
4	3	2	9	7	5	8	1	6
9	4	3	6	8	7	5	2	1
7	2	5	4	9	1	6	3	8
8	6	1	5	3	2	9	7	4
3	1	9	7	6	4	2	8	5
5	7	6	2	1	8	3	4	9
2	8	4	3	5	9	1	6	7

Puzzle #56 - Easy

4	9	3	2	8	6	5	1	7
8	1	6	7	9	5	3	4	2
7	5	2	4	1	3	9	6	8
5	2	1	8	6	7	4	9	3
9	7	4	3	5	2	6	8	1
6	3	8	9	4	1	2	7	5
2	8	5	6	7	4	1	3	9
1	6	7	5	3	9	8	2	4
3	4	9	1	2	8	7	5	6

Puzzle #57 - Easy

6	3	5	8	9	4	2	1	7
4	8	9	7	2	1	6	3	5
7	2	1	5	3	6	4	9	8
8	9	6	3	4	5	1	7	2
5	7	4	1	6	2	3	8	9
3	1	2	9	8	7	5	4	6
2	6	3	4	7	9	8	5	1
9	5	8	2	1	3	7	6	4
1	4	7	6	5	8	9	2	3

Puzzle #58 - Easy

3	8	7	9	1	5	2	6	4
9	5	6	2	8	4	1	7	3
1	4	2	7	6	3	9	5	8
4	1	9	5	3	8	6	2	7
5	2	3	4	7	6	8	1	9
7	6	8	1	2	9	4	3	5
6	7	4	3	9	1	5	8	2
8	3	5	6	4	2	7	9	1
2	9	1	8	5	7	3	4	6

Puzzle #59 - Easy

5	7	8	6	3	4	2	1	9
9	1	3	2	5	8	6	4	7
4	2	6	1	7	9	8	5	3
8	4	2	3	1	7	9	6	5
6	3	7	8	9	5	1	2	4
1	5	9	4	2	6	3	7	8
2	9	1	5	4	3	7	8	6
7	6	4	9	8	1	5	3	2
3	8	5	7	6	2	4	9	1

Puzzle #60 - Easy

3	5	4	6	9	8	2	1	7
9	7	8	2	1	3	6	5	4
1	2	6	4	7	5	9	3	8
8	4	9	5	3	6	7	2	1
7	1	2	9	8	4	5	6	3
5	6	3	1	2	7	8	4	9
4	9	7	3	6	2	1	8	5
6	8	5	7	4	1	3	9	2
2	3	1	8	5	9	4	7	6

Puzzle #61 - Easy

7	5	3	4	9	6	1	2	8
8	2	9	1	3	7	4	6	5
6	1	4	2	5	8	9	7	3
2	3	8	5	7	1	6	9	4
9	6	1	3	8	4	2	5	7
5	4	7	6	2	9	3	8	1
1	9	5	7	4	2	8	3	6
4	7	2	8	6	3	5	1	9
3	8	6	9	1	5	7	4	2

Puzzle #62 - Easy

5	2	9	6	8	4	7	3	1
7	3	4	1	9	5	8	6	2
8	1	6	2	7	3	5	4	9
1	9	7	8	4	6	3	2	5
2	5	8	3	1	9	6	7	4
4	6	3	5	2	7	9	1	8
6	4	1	7	5	8	2	9	3
9	7	5	4	3	2	1	8	6
3	8	2	9	6	1	4	5	7

Puzzle #63 - Easy

2	8	4	9	7	1	6	3	5
9	5	6	2	4	3	8	7	1
3	1	7	8	5	6	2	4	9
4	7	2	5	3	9	1	8	6
5	6	1	7	8	4	3	9	2
8	9	3	6	1	2	7	5	4
6	3	8	1	9	5	4	2	7
7	2	5	4	6	8	9	1	3
1	4	9	3	2	7	5	6	8

Puzzle #64 - Easy

8	7	5	9	3	1	6	2	4
4	6	9	2	7	8	1	3	5
1	3	2	4	5	6	8	9	7
6	4	8	5	9	3	2	7	1
9	2	3	7	1	4	5	8	6
7	5	1	6	8	2	3	4	9
5	8	7	1	2	9	4	6	3
3	9	6	8	4	5	7	1	2
2	1	4	3	6	7	9	5	8

Puzzle #65 - Easy

8	1	7	5	3	9	4	2	6
2	3	5	1	4	6	9	7	8
4	9	6	7	2	8	3	5	1
6	8	4	9	1	5	2	3	7
7	5	9	3	6	2	1	8	4
1	2	3	4	8	7	5	6	9
9	4	8	6	5	3	7	1	2
5	6	1	2	7	4	8	9	3
3	7	2	8	9	1	6	4	5

Puzzle #66 - Easy

1	9	4	6	7	3	5	2	8
5	7	2	9	4	8	6	3	1
6	8	3	5	1	2	7	9	4
8	1	6	7	3	9	4	5	2
7	3	5	4	2	6	1	8	9
4	2	9	8	5	1	3	7	6
2	5	7	1	9	4	8	6	3
3	6	1	2	8	7	9	4	5
9	4	8	3	6	5	2	1	7

Puzzle #67 - Easy

5	7	4	8	3	9	6	2	1
9	3	2	5	1	6	7	4	8
8	1	6	4	2	7	5	9	3
3	6	5	2	4	8	9	1	7
7	8	1	9	6	5	2	3	4
4	2	9	3	7	1	8	6	5
2	4	7	6	8	3	1	5	9
1	9	3	7	5	2	4	8	6
6	5	8	1	9	4	3	7	2

Puzzle #68 - Easy

3	6	5	9	8	4	2	7	1
1	9	4	2	7	5	8	3	6
2	8	7	3	1	6	9	5	4
9	4	8	5	2	7	6	1	3
5	1	2	6	3	8	7	4	9
6	7	3	1	4	9	5	8	2
8	5	1	4	9	2	3	6	7
7	3	9	8	6	1	4	2	5
4	2	6	7	5	3	1	9	8

Puzzle #69 - Easy

8	9	4	2	5	7	1	6	3
2	5	1	3	6	8	4	7	9
3	6	7	4	1	9	8	5	2
7	2	8	1	3	6	5	9	4
4	1	9	7	2	5	3	8	6
5	3	6	8	9	4	7	2	1
1	8	5	9	4	2	6	3	7
6	4	2	5	7	3	9	1	8
9	7	3	6	8	1	2	4	5

Puzzle #70 - Easy

6	5	3	9	1	7	2	4	8
8	1	7	2	3	4	9	6	5
2	9	4	8	6	5	3	7	1
4	7	2	1	5	9	6	8	3
5	8	6	3	7	2	1	9	4
9	3	1	4	8	6	7	5	2
7	4	5	6	2	1	8	3	9
1	6	8	5	9	3	4	2	7
3	2	9	7	4	8	5	1	6

Puzzle #71 - Easy

2	7	9	6	3	8	4	1	5
4	3	5	2	1	7	6	9	8
8	6	1	4	9	5	7	2	3
6	2	7	5	4	1	3	8	9
5	4	8	3	7	9	2	6	1
9	1	3	8	6	2	5	7	4
3	8	4	1	2	6	9	5	7
7	5	6	9	8	4	1	3	2
1	9	2	7	5	3	8	4	6

Puzzle #72 - Easy

1	8	9	7	3	5	6	4	2
3	7	6	4	2	9	1	8	5
4	5	2	8	1	6	9	7	3
8	6	3	2	5	7	4	1	9
2	1	7	9	4	8	5	3	6
9	4	5	3	6	1	7	2	8
5	2	8	1	9	4	3	6	7
7	9	4	6	8	3	2	5	1
6	3	1	5	7	2	8	9	4

Puzzle #73 - Easy

8	5	2	3	9	7	6	1	4
7	3	1	5	4	6	8	2	9
6	9	4	8	1	2	7	5	3
3	6	8	9	5	1	4	7	2
2	4	7	6	8	3	1	9	5
5	1	9	2	7	4	3	8	6
1	7	5	4	6	9	2	3	8
9	2	6	1	3	8	5	4	7
4	8	3	7	2	5	9	6	1

Puzzle #74 - Easy

6	7	4	3	2	1	8	9	5
9	3	2	8	4	5	6	1	7
5	1	8	9	7	6	3	4	2
7	4	3	5	8	9	2	6	1
1	9	5	4	6	2	7	8	3
8	2	6	7	1	3	4	5	9
2	8	9	6	5	7	1	3	4
3	6	1	2	9	4	5	7	8
4	5	7	1	3	8	9	2	6

Puzzle #75 - Easy

5	8	4	3	9	7	1	6	2
9	3	1	8	2	6	4	7	5
6	7	2	5	1	4	9	8	3
3	4	8	1	6	2	7	5	9
7	6	5	9	4	8	2	3	1
1	2	9	7	3	5	6	4	8
4	5	3	2	7	1	8	9	6
2	9	7	6	8	3	5	1	4
8	1	6	4	5	9	3	2	7

Puzzle #76 - Easy

1	5	9	3	7	8	4	2	6
6	3	7	1	2	4	8	9	5
8	4	2	9	6	5	3	1	7
7	6	4	5	3	2	9	8	1
2	9	1	7	8	6	5	4	3
3	8	5	4	9	1	7	6	2
4	2	6	8	5	3	1	7	9
5	7	8	2	1	9	6	3	4
9	1	3	6	4	7	2	5	8

Puzzle #77 - Easy

5	8	3	2	6	9	4	1	7
4	1	9	7	8	5	6	3	2
6	2	7	4	3	1	9	8	5
1	4	2	9	7	8	5	6	3
3	9	5	1	4	6	7	2	8
7	6	8	5	2	3	1	9	4
8	7	6	3	1	4	2	5	9
2	5	1	8	9	7	3	4	6
9	3	4	6	5	2	8	7	1

Puzzle #78 - Easy

2	3	8	9	6	4	5	7	1
9	6	1	5	2	7	3	8	4
5	4	7	8	3	1	6	2	9
1	9	5	3	8	6	7	4	2
3	8	6	4	7	2	9	1	5
4	7	2	1	5	9	8	6	3
7	5	3	2	1	8	4	9	6
8	2	9	6	4	5	1	3	7
6	1	4	7	9	3	2	5	8

Puzzle #79 - Easy

6	7	3	8	5	1	9	4	2
4	2	1	3	9	7	6	5	8
8	9	5	4	6	2	3	1	7
1	5	7	6	3	4	8	2	9
9	6	4	2	7	8	5	3	1
3	8	2	9	1	5	7	6	4
7	1	8	5	2	3	4	9	6
5	4	9	1	8	6	2	7	3
2	3	6	7	4	9	1	8	5

Puzzle #80 - Easy

2	6	4	9	1	5	3	8	7
1	9	7	8	2	3	6	5	4
3	8	5	4	7	6	2	9	1
5	1	3	6	4	2	8	7	9
4	7	8	3	9	1	5	6	2
6	2	9	5	8	7	1	4	3
8	4	6	2	3	9	7	1	5
9	3	1	7	5	8	4	2	6
7	5	2	1	6	4	9	3	8

Puzzle #81 - Easy

1	6	4	8	7	5	3	9	2
2	8	9	1	3	4	6	7	5
7	3	5	9	6	2	1	4	8
4	5	6	3	2	1	7	8	9
9	2	3	7	4	8	5	6	1
8	7	1	5	9	6	2	3	4
3	1	2	4	8	7	9	5	6
6	9	8	2	5	3	4	1	7
5	4	7	6	1	9	8	2	3

Puzzle #82 - Easy

1	3	5	4	2	7	8	6	9
2	7	9	6	8	5	1	3	4
4	6	8	9	3	1	7	2	5
9	5	6	7	1	3	2	4	8
3	8	4	2	9	6	5	7	1
7	1	2	8	5	4	3	9	6
5	4	1	3	6	2	9	8	7
8	2	7	1	4	9	6	5	3
6	9	3	5	7	8	4	1	2

Puzzle #83 - Easy

6	4	2	3	5	8	7	9	1
8	5	7	9	1	2	3	4	6
3	9	1	7	4	6	5	8	2
2	8	4	5	6	9	1	7	3
7	6	3	4	2	1	9	5	8
9	1	5	8	7	3	2	6	4
4	7	6	2	3	5	8	1	9
1	2	9	6	8	7	4	3	5
5	3	8	1	9	4	6	2	7

Puzzle #84 - Easy

5	7	8	1	3	9	6	4	2
2	3	1	6	5	4	8	7	9
9	6	4	8	7	2	1	5	3
3	2	9	4	1	7	5	6	8
8	4	6	3	9	5	2	1	7
1	5	7	2	8	6	3	9	4
7	8	5	9	2	1	4	3	6
4	1	2	7	6	3	9	8	5
6	9	3	5	4	8	7	2	1

Puzzle #85 - Easy

9	2	3	8	4	7	5	1	6
7	4	5	6	9	1	8	2	3
8	6	1	5	3	2	9	7	4
6	1	8	4	2	3	7	5	9
4	9	2	7	6	5	3	8	1
5	3	7	1	8	9	6	4	2
2	5	9	3	1	8	4	6	7
3	7	6	2	5	4	1	9	8
1	8	4	9	7	6	2	3	5

Puzzle #86 - Easy

4	7	2	6	8	3	1	9	5
1	9	5	2	7	4	3	8	6
6	8	3	9	5	1	4	7	2
2	6	9	1	3	8	5	4	7
8	3	4	7	2	5	9	6	1
7	5	1	4	6	9	2	3	8
3	1	7	5	4	6	8	2	9
9	4	6	8	1	2	7	5	3
5	2	8	3	9	7	6	1	4

Puzzle #87 - Easy

7	2	1	3	9	6	8	4	5
4	3	6	5	8	7	1	2	9
9	8	5	2	1	4	3	6	7
2	1	7	6	4	8	5	9	3
3	9	4	7	5	1	6	8	2
5	6	8	9	2	3	7	1	4
6	4	2	8	7	5	9	3	1
8	7	9	1	3	2	4	5	6
1	5	3	4	6	9	2	7	8

Puzzle #88 - Easy

4	7	5	8	3	2	6	1	9
2	9	3	5	6	1	8	7	4
6	8	1	9	4	7	5	2	3
3	5	7	6	2	4	1	9	8
9	4	2	3	1	8	7	5	6
1	6	8	7	9	5	4	3	2
8	1	4	2	5	3	9	6	7
7	3	6	1	8	9	2	4	5
5	2	9	4	7	6	3	8	1

Puzzle #89 - Easy

7	5	1	2	6	4	3	9	8
8	4	6	7	9	3	5	2	1
2	3	9	1	5	8	4	7	6
5	9	7	3	8	1	2	6	4
1	8	4	9	2	6	7	3	5
6	2	3	5	4	7	8	1	9
4	1	8	6	3	2	9	5	7
9	6	2	8	7	5	1	4	3
3	7	5	4	1	9	6	8	2

Puzzle #90 - Easy

2	8	9	6	4	5	7	1	3
1	6	4	7	9	3	8	2	5
5	7	3	2	1	8	6	4	9
3	2	8	9	6	4	1	5	7
4	5	7	8	3	1	9	6	2
6	9	1	5	2	7	4	3	8
8	3	6	4	7	2	5	9	1
7	4	2	1	5	9	3	8	6
9	1	5	3	8	6	2	7	4

Puzzle #91 - Easy

9	3	5	6	7	1	8	2	4
4	7	6	8	5	2	1	3	9
8	2	1	4	9	3	7	5	6
6	8	2	9	3	4	5	1	7
3	1	4	5	2	7	9	6	8
5	9	7	1	6	8	3	4	2
2	5	3	7	4	9	6	8	1
7	6	8	2	1	5	4	9	3
1	4	9	3	8	6	2	7	5

Puzzle #92 - Easy

8	5	9	6	4	2	3	1	7
4	1	2	9	3	7	6	5	8
6	3	7	5	8	1	9	4	2
2	6	3	4	7	9	1	8	5
5	9	4	8	1	6	2	7	3
7	8	1	2	5	3	4	9	6
3	2	8	1	9	5	7	6	4
1	7	5	3	6	4	8	2	9
9	4	6	7	2	8	5	3	1

Puzzle #93 - Easy

3	1	8	9	5	2	6	7	4
2	5	4	6	7	3	9	8	1
9	7	6	4	8	1	3	5	2
1	8	9	7	3	5	4	2	6
4	2	3	8	1	6	5	9	7
7	6	5	2	9	4	8	1	3
5	3	2	1	6	8	7	4	9
6	9	1	5	4	7	2	3	8
8	4	7	3	2	9	1	6	5

Puzzle #94 - Easy

9	3	2	7	4	8	6	5	1
8	1	7	5	9	6	3	2	4
4	6	5	3	2	1	8	7	9
2	9	8	1	3	4	7	6	5
7	5	3	9	6	2	4	1	8
1	4	6	8	7	5	9	3	2
5	7	4	6	1	9	2	8	3
3	2	1	4	8	7	5	9	6
6	8	9	2	5	3	1	4	7

Puzzle #95 - Easy

2	3	9	1	5	6	7	8	4
4	5	7	2	8	3	1	6	9
6	1	8	7	9	4	2	5	3
5	9	2	6	4	7	8	3	1
8	4	1	3	2	5	6	9	7
7	6	3	9	1	8	4	2	5
1	8	6	5	7	9	3	4	2
9	2	4	8	3	1	5	7	6
3	7	5	4	6	2	9	1	8

Puzzle #96 - Easy

5	4	3	7	1	6	8	2	9
1	6	9	5	8	2	4	3	7
7	8	2	3	4	9	1	6	5
4	3	8	9	2	5	6	7	1
2	7	1	4	6	8	9	5	3
6	9	5	1	3	7	2	4	8
8	1	6	2	7	3	5	9	4
3	5	4	6	9	1	7	8	2
9	2	7	8	5	4	3	1	6

Puzzle #97 - Easy

7	2	6	3	9	8	1	5	4
3	1	9	5	4	7	2	8	6
8	4	5	2	1	6	9	3	7
1	6	8	7	3	2	5	4	9
5	3	4	6	8	9	7	2	1
9	7	2	4	5	1	8	6	3
4	8	3	9	7	5	6	1	2
6	5	7	1	2	3	4	9	8
2	9	1	8	6	4	3	7	5

Puzzle #98 - Easy

9	5	6	2	8	4	7	3	1
3	8	4	6	1	7	5	2	9
7	1	2	9	3	5	8	6	4
6	9	1	4	7	3	2	8	5
8	2	7	1	5	6	9	4	3
4	3	5	8	9	2	6	1	7
1	6	8	5	4	9	3	7	2
5	4	3	7	2	8	1	9	6
2	7	9	3	6	1	4	5	8

Puzzle #99 - Easy

3	9	4	2	5	6	7	8	1
7	8	6	4	1	3	5	2	9
5	2	1	7	9	8	4	3	6
6	7	8	3	2	5	9	1	4
9	3	5	6	4	1	2	7	8
4	1	2	8	7	9	6	5	3
8	5	3	9	6	2	1	4	7
1	4	9	5	8	7	3	6	2
2	6	7	1	3	4	8	9	5

Puzzle #100 - Easy

2	3	8	4	5	6	9	7	1
1	5	9	7	8	3	6	4	2
7	6	4	1	9	2	8	5	3
4	2	6	9	7	8	1	3	5
8	7	5	3	4	1	2	9	6
9	1	3	2	6	5	7	8	4
3	9	2	5	1	7	4	6	8
6	4	1	8	3	9	5	2	7
5	8	7	6	2	4	3	1	9

Puzzle #1 - Medium

2	8	7	6	4	1	9	3	5
1	9	3	8	5	2	6	7	4
5	6	4	9	7	3	8	2	1
8	4	6	5	3	9	7	1	2
9	2	5	7	1	8	3	4	6
3	7	1	2	6	4	5	9	8
7	1	9	4	8	6	2	5	3
6	3	2	1	9	5	4	8	7
4	5	8	3	2	7	1	6	9

Puzzle #2 - Medium

1	3	4	7	8	5	2	9	6
2	5	6	1	9	4	3	8	7
9	8	7	2	3	6	5	4	1
6	4	5	8	1	9	7	3	2
3	9	1	5	2	7	4	6	8
8	7	2	4	6	3	1	5	9
4	6	9	3	7	2	8	1	5
5	2	8	9	4	1	6	7	3
7	1	3	6	5	8	9	2	4

Puzzle #3 - Medium

7	3	5	4	9	1	8	6	2
4	2	8	7	6	5	9	1	3
6	9	1	8	2	3	4	5	7
9	5	3	2	4	6	7	8	1
1	8	4	3	7	9	6	2	5
2	7	6	1	5	8	3	9	4
8	4	9	5	3	2	1	7	6
5	1	7	6	8	4	2	3	9
3	6	2	9	1	7	5	4	8

Puzzle #4 - Medium

9	6	4	8	3	5	2	7	1
8	7	3	2	1	4	5	9	6
2	1	5	9	6	7	4	3	8
7	9	1	6	5	8	3	2	4
4	2	6	3	7	1	9	8	5
3	5	8	4	9	2	6	1	7
5	8	2	1	4	9	7	6	3
1	3	7	5	2	6	8	4	9
6	4	9	7	8	3	1	5	2

Puzzle #5 - Medium

1	9	5	4	6	3	2	8	7
7	2	3	8	1	9	5	6	4
4	8	6	5	2	7	1	3	9
9	4	2	6	5	8	3	7	1
8	5	1	3	7	2	9	4	6
6	3	7	9	4	1	8	5	2
2	6	9	7	8	5	4	1	3
5	1	4	2	3	6	7	9	8
3	7	8	1	9	4	6	2	5

Puzzle #6 - Medium

3	6	2	1	5	7	8	9	4
7	5	4	9	8	6	2	1	3
8	1	9	2	4	3	6	7	5
6	4	7	8	3	2	9	5	1
9	8	1	4	7	5	3	2	6
2	3	5	6	1	9	4	8	7
4	7	8	3	9	1	5	6	2
5	2	3	7	6	8	1	4	9
1	9	6	5	2	4	7	3	8

Puzzle #7 - Medium

7	1	2	6	4	8	9	3	5
5	9	8	1	7	3	4	6	2
3	4	6	5	2	9	8	1	7
8	2	1	4	6	5	3	7	9
6	7	4	3	9	1	2	5	8
9	3	5	7	8	2	1	4	6
2	5	3	9	1	7	6	8	4
4	8	7	2	3	6	5	9	1
1	6	9	8	5	4	7	2	3

Puzzle #8 - Medium

4	6	9	1	2	5	7	3	8
8	5	2	7	3	6	1	9	4
3	1	7	8	9	4	5	6	2
9	7	1	3	4	2	6	8	5
5	3	8	6	7	1	4	2	9
2	4	6	9	5	8	3	1	7
6	9	4	2	1	7	8	5	3
7	8	3	5	6	9	2	4	1
1	2	5	4	8	3	9	7	6

Puzzle #9 - Medium

3	5	4	9	8	2	6	1	7
2	6	8	1	7	5	3	9	4
1	7	9	4	3	6	2	5	8
8	4	5	6	2	9	7	3	1
6	3	7	8	4	1	5	2	9
9	2	1	7	5	3	4	8	6
7	8	3	5	1	4	9	6	2
4	9	2	3	6	8	1	7	5
5	1	6	2	9	7	8	4	3

Puzzle #10 - Medium

6	2	4	1	3	7	8	9	5
3	5	9	6	8	4	2	1	7
1	7	8	5	9	2	6	4	3
5	8	2	3	1	9	4	7	6
7	9	3	4	5	6	1	2	8
4	6	1	7	2	8	5	3	9
2	3	7	8	4	5	9	6	1
8	4	6	9	7	1	3	5	2
9	1	5	2	6	3	7	8	4

Puzzle #11 - Medium

3	5	7	2	8	4	1	9	6
9	1	4	3	5	6	2	7	8
2	6	8	7	1	9	3	4	5
7	2	5	4	3	8	9	6	1
6	4	3	9	2	1	8	5	7
8	9	1	6	7	5	4	2	3
1	3	2	5	4	7	6	8	9
5	8	9	1	6	2	7	3	4
4	7	6	8	9	3	5	1	2

Puzzle #12 - Medium

5	2	6	4	7	9	8	1	3
7	3	1	5	8	6	9	2	4
8	4	9	3	2	1	6	5	7
1	5	8	9	6	4	7	3	2
2	7	3	1	5	8	4	9	6
9	6	4	7	3	2	5	8	1
3	1	5	8	4	7	2	6	9
4	9	2	6	1	5	3	7	8
6	8	7	2	9	3	1	4	5

Puzzle #13 - Medium

5	2	7	1	3	9	4	8	6
4	6	3	2	8	7	1	9	5
8	1	9	5	6	4	7	2	3
6	5	8	3	7	1	9	4	2
9	4	1	8	5	2	6	3	7
3	7	2	9	4	6	8	5	1
7	8	5	4	1	3	2	6	9
1	9	4	6	2	5	3	7	8
2	3	6	7	9	8	5	1	4

Puzzle #14 - Medium

8	3	6	5	7	1	9	4	2
7	2	9	3	4	8	1	5	6
4	5	1	2	6	9	8	7	3
9	6	2	1	3	7	4	8	5
3	7	5	6	8	4	2	9	1
1	8	4	9	2	5	3	6	7
2	9	8	7	1	6	5	3	4
6	4	3	8	5	2	7	1	9
5	1	7	4	9	3	6	2	8

Puzzle #15 - Medium

3	2	6	5	7	4	8	1	9
4	8	7	9	1	6	3	5	2
9	5	1	2	3	8	4	7	6
8	9	4	7	5	1	6	2	3
6	7	5	3	4	2	1	9	8
2	1	3	6	8	9	5	4	7
1	4	9	8	6	7	2	3	5
7	3	8	4	2	5	9	6	1
5	6	2	1	9	3	7	8	4

Puzzle #16 - Medium

6	2	1	5	9	8	7	4	3
9	3	8	4	6	7	5	2	1
4	7	5	1	2	3	6	9	8
7	5	6	8	1	9	4	3	2
3	8	4	7	5	2	9	1	6
2	1	9	6	3	4	8	7	5
8	4	2	3	7	5	1	6	9
5	6	3	9	4	1	2	8	7
1	9	7	2	8	6	3	5	4

Puzzle #17 - Medium

5	7	4	8	6	9	3	2	1
1	2	6	3	7	4	8	9	5
8	3	9	1	5	2	7	6	4
4	8	3	6	9	1	2	5	7
9	1	2	5	8	7	4	3	6
6	5	7	2	4	3	9	1	8
7	9	1	4	3	5	6	8	2
2	4	8	9	1	6	5	7	3
3	6	5	7	2	8	1	4	9

Puzzle #18 - Medium

3	5	8	9	2	1	6	4	7
6	1	4	5	7	8	9	2	3
2	7	9	3	6	4	1	8	5
7	4	2	6	8	9	3	5	1
9	6	5	2	1	3	8	7	4
1	8	3	4	5	7	2	6	9
5	2	1	7	3	6	4	9	8
8	9	6	1	4	5	7	3	2
4	3	7	8	9	2	5	1	6

Puzzle #19 - Medium

7	8	6	5	4	1	2	9	3
2	9	4	8	7	3	6	1	5
5	1	3	9	6	2	8	4	7
6	2	5	3	1	8	4	7	9
9	4	8	7	5	6	3	2	1
1	3	7	4	2	9	5	8	6
3	7	2	6	9	4	1	5	8
4	6	9	1	8	5	7	3	2
8	5	1	2	3	7	9	6	4

Puzzle #20 - Medium

5	6	7	2	3	1	8	9	4
1	8	3	7	4	9	5	6	2
2	9	4	8	5	6	7	1	3
4	1	5	9	2	3	6	7	8
7	3	8	1	6	5	4	2	9
6	2	9	4	8	7	3	5	1
3	7	2	6	9	4	1	8	5
9	4	6	5	1	8	2	3	7
8	5	1	3	7	2	9	4	6

Puzzle #21 - Medium

6	7	1	4	5	3	9	2	8
3	4	9	8	6	2	1	5	7
2	8	5	9	7	1	4	6	3
8	3	4	6	1	5	2	7	9
9	2	6	3	8	7	5	4	1
1	5	7	2	9	4	3	8	6
5	9	2	7	3	6	8	1	4
7	1	3	5	4	8	6	9	2
4	6	8	1	2	9	7	3	5

Puzzle #22 - Medium

1	6	8	9	4	3	7	5	2
4	5	7	2	8	6	9	3	1
2	9	3	7	1	5	8	4	6
9	4	6	3	2	8	5	1	7
7	3	1	5	9	4	2	6	8
5	8	2	6	7	1	3	9	4
3	7	9	4	6	2	1	8	5
6	1	5	8	3	7	4	2	9
8	2	4	1	5	9	6	7	3

Puzzle #23 - Medium

5	4	6	8	3	9	1	7	2
7	8	2	6	1	4	5	3	9
9	1	3	2	5	7	6	8	4
1	5	4	7	2	8	9	6	3
2	7	9	3	6	1	4	5	8
6	3	8	9	4	5	2	1	7
4	6	7	5	8	2	3	9	1
8	2	5	1	9	3	7	4	6
3	9	1	4	7	6	8	2	5

Puzzle #24 - Medium

2	1	4	8	9	6	7	3	5
3	9	7	1	5	4	2	6	8
5	6	8	2	3	7	1	4	9
8	2	9	7	4	5	3	1	6
4	3	1	9	6	8	5	7	2
6	7	5	3	1	2	9	8	4
9	8	2	4	7	3	6	5	1
1	5	3	6	8	9	4	2	7
7	4	6	5	2	1	8	9	3

Puzzle #25 - Medium

7	8	3	4	6	9	1	2	5
1	4	9	8	5	2	7	3	6
5	2	6	3	1	7	8	9	4
3	7	1	2	4	6	9	5	8
4	9	2	5	3	8	6	7	1
6	5	8	9	7	1	3	4	2
2	1	4	7	8	3	5	6	9
9	6	7	1	2	5	4	8	3
8	3	5	6	9	4	2	1	7

Puzzle #26 - Medium

2	9	3	1	8	6	4	7	5
1	8	7	2	4	5	3	6	9
5	4	6	7	3	9	2	1	8
4	3	8	6	1	7	9	5	2
9	7	2	4	5	3	1	8	6
6	1	5	9	2	8	7	3	4
8	2	4	3	6	1	5	9	7
7	5	1	8	9	2	6	4	3
3	6	9	5	7	4	8	2	1

Puzzle #27 - Medium

9	2	6	3	1	7	5	4	8
1	4	8	2	9	5	7	3	6
3	5	7	8	6	4	1	2	9
2	8	9	1	7	6	4	5	3
5	7	1	9	4	3	8	6	2
6	3	4	5	8	2	9	7	1
4	1	5	6	2	9	3	8	7
8	6	3	7	5	1	2	9	4
7	9	2	4	3	8	6	1	5

Puzzle #28 - Medium

1	5	4	3	2	9	6	8	7
9	3	7	1	8	6	5	4	2
8	2	6	4	7	5	3	1	9
6	7	3	8	5	1	2	9	4
4	1	5	2	9	7	8	3	6
2	9	8	6	3	4	7	5	1
3	8	1	9	6	2	4	7	5
7	4	2	5	1	8	9	6	3
5	6	9	7	4	3	1	2	8

Puzzle #29 - Medium

9	4	7	1	5	8	3	6	2
3	1	5	6	4	2	9	7	8
8	6	2	3	9	7	1	4	5
5	7	9	2	6	1	8	3	4
6	2	3	9	8	4	5	1	7
4	8	1	7	3	5	2	9	6
2	9	4	8	7	3	6	5	1
1	5	6	4	2	9	7	8	3
7	3	8	5	1	6	4	2	9

Puzzle #30 - Medium

2	5	7	3	1	9	6	4	8
6	4	3	8	2	7	5	1	9
1	8	9	6	5	4	3	7	2
3	2	6	9	7	8	4	5	1
9	1	4	2	6	5	8	3	7
8	7	5	1	4	3	9	2	6
7	3	2	4	9	6	1	8	5
4	9	1	5	8	2	7	6	3
5	6	8	7	3	1	2	9	4

Puzzle #31 - Medium

2	8	3	7	4	1	9	5	6
6	1	4	9	3	5	2	7	8
9	5	7	2	6	8	3	4	1
3	7	5	4	2	6	1	8	9
8	4	6	1	9	7	5	2	3
1	2	9	5	8	3	4	6	7
4	9	1	8	7	2	6	3	5
7	6	2	3	5	9	8	1	4
5	3	8	6	1	4	7	9	2

Puzzle #32 - Medium

8	9	6	1	3	5	7	2	4
2	1	5	7	6	4	3	9	8
7	3	4	9	2	8	1	5	6
1	2	3	6	5	7	4	8	9
4	5	7	8	9	2	6	1	3
6	8	9	4	1	3	2	7	5
3	7	2	5	8	6	9	4	1
9	6	8	2	4	1	5	3	7
5	4	1	3	7	9	8	6	2

Puzzle #33 - Medium

8	4	3	1	7	2	9	6	5
2	6	1	5	9	4	3	8	7
5	9	7	6	3	8	2	1	4
1	8	4	7	2	9	5	3	6
7	2	9	3	6	5	1	4	8
6	3	5	8	4	1	7	9	2
3	5	2	4	1	6	8	7	9
9	1	6	2	8	7	4	5	3
4	7	8	9	5	3	6	2	1

Puzzle #34 - Medium

8	6	2	4	1	9	5	7	3
4	5	7	8	3	2	1	6	9
9	1	3	7	5	6	8	4	2
7	8	1	2	6	4	3	9	5
6	2	5	3	9	7	4	1	8
3	9	4	1	8	5	6	2	7
1	7	6	5	2	3	9	8	4
2	3	9	6	4	8	7	5	1
5	4	8	9	7	1	2	3	6

Puzzle #35 - Medium

1	2	5	6	7	4	8	9	3
8	6	4	9	3	1	7	2	5
3	7	9	2	8	5	6	1	4
9	3	7	8	4	6	1	5	2
6	4	2	5	1	9	3	8	7
5	1	8	3	2	7	4	6	9
7	5	3	1	6	2	9	4	8
4	9	6	7	5	8	2	3	1
2	8	1	4	9	3	5	7	6

Puzzle #36 - Medium

2	7	1	8	3	6	4	9	5
4	8	5	9	7	2	6	3	1
9	3	6	4	5	1	2	7	8
6	4	8	3	1	9	5	2	7
1	2	7	6	4	5	3	8	9
5	9	3	2	8	7	1	6	4
8	5	2	1	9	3	7	4	6
3	1	9	7	6	4	8	5	2
7	6	4	5	2	8	9	1	3

Puzzle #37 - Medium

3	2	6	7	9	1	5	4	8
8	9	4	2	5	3	1	7	6
5	7	1	4	6	8	2	3	9
4	8	2	5	7	6	9	1	3
6	1	9	3	8	2	4	5	7
7	5	3	1	4	9	8	6	2
9	3	5	6	2	4	7	8	1
2	6	7	8	1	5	3	9	4
1	4	8	9	3	7	6	2	5

Puzzle #38 - Medium

2	1	5	8	3	9	6	4	7
9	8	6	5	7	4	2	1	3
4	3	7	1	2	6	9	5	8
1	6	9	4	8	3	5	7	2
3	2	4	6	5	7	1	8	9
7	5	8	9	1	2	3	6	4
8	7	2	3	6	5	4	9	1
6	9	1	2	4	8	7	3	5
5	4	3	7	9	1	8	2	6

Puzzle #39 - Medium

7	1	2	6	4	5	8	9	3
8	6	4	3	1	9	2	7	5
3	5	9	2	8	7	6	4	1
9	3	1	7	6	4	5	2	8
2	8	5	1	9	3	4	6	7
4	7	6	5	2	8	1	3	9
5	4	8	9	7	2	3	1	6
6	9	3	4	5	1	7	8	2
1	2	7	8	3	6	9	5	4

Puzzle #40 - Medium

1	8	6	3	4	5	9	7	2
2	9	5	8	6	7	4	3	1
3	4	7	9	1	2	6	8	5
9	5	8	2	7	6	1	4	3
4	7	2	1	3	8	5	6	9
6	3	1	5	9	4	8	2	7
7	1	4	6	2	9	3	5	8
5	6	9	7	8	3	2	1	4
8	2	3	4	5	1	7	9	6

Puzzle #41 - Medium

8	9	2	4	3	5	7	1	6
3	4	6	9	1	7	8	5	2
7	1	5	8	2	6	4	9	3
4	8	1	7	6	3	9	2	5
5	7	3	1	9	2	6	8	4
2	6	9	5	8	4	1	3	7
1	5	4	3	7	8	2	6	9
9	2	7	6	5	1	3	4	8
6	3	8	2	4	9	5	7	1

Puzzle #42 - Medium

5	1	6	7	9	2	4	3	8
7	8	3	4	1	5	6	2	9
4	9	2	8	6	3	7	5	1
1	7	9	6	3	4	5	8	2
2	6	8	5	7	1	9	4	3
3	5	4	2	8	9	1	7	6
9	2	1	3	5	7	8	6	4
8	4	5	9	2	6	3	1	7
6	3	7	1	4	8	2	9	5

Puzzle #43 - Medium

2	4	8	3	6	1	5	7	9
6	9	3	5	7	4	8	1	2
5	1	7	8	9	2	6	3	4
8	7	1	2	4	5	3	9	6
4	6	5	7	3	9	2	8	1
9	3	2	1	8	6	4	5	7
3	8	4	6	1	7	9	2	5
7	2	9	4	5	3	1	6	8
1	5	6	9	2	8	7	4	3

Puzzle #44 - Medium

2	9	3	8	6	4	1	7	5
5	8	4	1	9	7	6	2	3
1	6	7	3	5	2	4	9	8
8	2	6	9	4	1	3	5	7
4	7	5	2	8	3	9	1	6
9	3	1	6	7	5	2	8	4
7	1	8	4	2	6	5	3	9
3	4	9	5	1	8	7	6	2
6	5	2	7	3	9	8	4	1

Puzzle #45 - Medium

8	6	4	7	5	2	1	9	3
3	5	9	4	1	6	8	7	2
7	1	2	9	3	8	4	5	6
4	7	6	3	9	1	2	8	5
2	8	5	6	7	4	9	3	1
9	3	1	2	8	5	6	4	7
1	2	7	5	4	9	3	6	8
6	9	3	8	2	7	5	1	4
5	4	8	1	6	3	7	2	9

Puzzle #46 - Medium

6	1	5	4	9	2	8	7	3
7	3	8	6	5	1	4	2	9
4	9	2	8	3	7	5	1	6
1	5	4	2	6	8	3	9	7
3	2	6	7	4	9	1	5	8
9	8	7	5	1	3	6	4	2
5	7	1	3	2	6	9	8	4
2	6	9	1	8	4	7	3	5
8	4	3	9	7	5	2	6	1

Puzzle #47 - Medium

2	8	9	6	3	4	7	5	1
4	5	7	8	1	2	3	6	9
1	3	6	5	7	9	8	2	4
5	2	4	3	9	6	1	8	7
9	7	3	2	8	1	5	4	6
6	1	8	4	5	7	2	9	3
7	6	1	9	2	5	4	3	8
8	9	2	7	4	3	6	1	5
3	4	5	1	6	8	9	7	2

Puzzle #48 - Medium

4	1	3	8	9	6	7	5	2
6	5	7	2	3	1	8	9	4
8	9	2	5	7	4	1	3	6
7	6	4	1	5	2	9	8	3
1	3	5	9	6	8	2	4	7
9	2	8	3	4	7	5	6	1
2	4	1	6	8	9	3	7	5
5	8	6	7	2	3	4	1	9
3	7	9	4	1	5	6	2	8

Puzzle #49 - Medium

4	3	8	6	9	7	1	5	2
5	9	6	1	2	4	7	3	8
2	7	1	3	8	5	6	4	9
3	2	4	5	6	8	9	1	7
6	1	7	9	4	2	5	8	3
9	8	5	7	3	1	2	6	4
7	6	3	4	1	9	8	2	5
1	5	2	8	7	3	4	9	6
8	4	9	2	5	6	3	7	1

Puzzle #50 - Medium

8	3	5	4	6	7	9	2	1
9	7	1	5	2	3	6	4	8
2	6	4	1	8	9	5	7	3
6	8	2	3	4	1	7	5	9
4	1	7	9	5	6	3	8	2
3	5	9	2	7	8	4	1	6
1	4	6	7	9	2	8	3	5
7	2	8	6	3	5	1	9	4
5	9	3	8	1	4	2	6	7

Puzzle #51 - Medium

5	7	6	4	8	2	3	9	1
1	4	9	7	5	3	2	8	6
3	8	2	6	1	9	7	4	5
9	3	7	1	4	8	5	6	2
6	2	4	9	3	5	1	7	8
8	1	5	2	6	7	4	3	9
4	6	8	5	7	1	9	2	3
2	5	3	8	9	4	6	1	7
7	9	1	3	2	6	8	5	4

Puzzle #52 - Medium

7	3	5	4	9	1	8	6	2
6	9	1	8	2	3	4	5	7
4	2	8	7	6	5	9	1	3
5	1	7	6	8	4	2	3	9
8	4	9	5	3	2	1	7	6
3	6	2	9	1	7	5	4	8
1	8	4	3	7	9	6	2	5
2	7	6	1	5	8	3	9	4
9	5	3	2	4	6	7	8	1

Puzzle #53 - Medium

2	9	4	8	3	5	1	6	7
8	5	6	1	7	9	2	3	4
1	7	3	6	4	2	8	9	5
7	6	9	5	2	1	3	4	8
4	1	2	3	8	7	9	5	6
5	3	8	4	9	6	7	2	1
6	2	5	7	1	3	4	8	9
9	4	1	2	5	8	6	7	3
3	8	7	9	6	4	5	1	2

Puzzle #54 - Medium

6	1	9	4	5	8	7	2	3
5	2	3	7	1	9	6	8	4
8	4	7	6	3	2	5	9	1
4	3	6	9	2	5	8	1	7
9	5	8	3	7	1	4	6	2
1	7	2	8	4	6	9	3	5
7	6	4	1	9	3	2	5	8
2	8	1	5	6	4	3	7	9
3	9	5	2	8	7	1	4	6

Puzzle #55 - Medium

4	6	9	1	2	3	8	5	7
2	1	8	6	5	7	3	9	4
7	3	5	8	9	4	2	6	1
5	8	1	9	4	6	7	2	3
6	2	4	7	3	8	9	1	5
9	7	3	2	1	5	6	4	8
3	9	7	4	6	1	5	8	2
8	4	6	5	7	2	1	3	9
1	5	2	3	8	9	4	7	6

Puzzle #56 - Medium

5	8	1	6	2	4	3	7	9
3	7	6	5	9	1	8	2	4
9	2	4	3	7	8	6	1	5
7	1	5	2	8	3	9	4	6
4	9	3	7	1	6	5	8	2
8	6	2	9	4	5	7	3	1
6	4	8	1	5	7	2	9	3
1	3	9	8	6	2	4	5	7
2	5	7	4	3	9	1	6	8

Puzzle #57 - Medium

9	8	3	7	4	5	6	1	2
4	5	6	2	1	8	3	9	7
1	7	2	3	9	6	4	8	5
5	3	8	6	2	1	7	4	9
2	1	9	4	5	7	8	6	3
6	4	7	9	8	3	2	5	1
7	6	1	5	3	4	9	2	8
3	2	5	8	6	9	1	7	4
8	9	4	1	7	2	5	3	6

Puzzle #58 - Medium

8	2	7	6	1	4	5	3	9
4	6	5	8	3	9	1	7	2
1	3	9	2	5	7	6	8	4
6	7	4	5	8	2	3	9	1
9	1	3	4	7	6	8	2	5
2	5	8	1	9	3	7	4	6
3	8	6	9	4	5	2	1	7
5	4	1	7	2	8	9	6	3
7	9	2	3	6	1	4	5	8

Puzzle #59 - Medium

7	8	3	5	6	1	4	2	9
9	1	5	4	8	2	6	7	3
2	4	6	9	3	7	1	8	5
3	9	4	8	1	6	7	5	2
6	2	8	7	4	5	9	3	1
5	7	1	3	2	9	8	4	6
4	5	9	1	7	3	2	6	8
1	6	7	2	5	8	3	9	4
8	3	2	6	9	4	5	1	7

Puzzle #60 - Medium

4	8	7	6	1	9	5	3	2
3	2	6	4	7	5	1	8	9
9	5	1	8	3	2	7	4	6
2	1	3	9	8	6	4	5	7
8	9	4	1	5	7	2	6	3
6	7	5	2	4	3	9	1	8
5	6	2	3	9	1	8	7	4
7	3	8	5	2	4	6	9	1
1	4	9	7	6	8	3	2	5

Puzzle #61 - Medium

8	9	1	5	6	7	2	4	3
7	2	5	8	4	3	6	9	1
6	4	3	1	9	2	5	8	7
9	1	4	6	3	5	7	2	8
2	6	8	9	7	1	4	3	5
3	5	7	4	2	8	9	1	6
1	3	2	7	5	4	8	6	9
4	7	6	3	8	9	1	5	2
5	8	9	2	1	6	3	7	4

Puzzle #62 - Medium

3	2	1	4	8	9	5	7	6
5	8	6	3	7	1	2	4	9
4	7	9	2	5	6	1	3	8
7	3	2	6	9	4	8	1	5
9	6	4	5	1	8	3	2	7
1	5	8	7	2	3	9	6	4
6	1	5	9	4	2	7	8	3
2	9	3	8	6	7	4	5	1
8	4	7	1	3	5	6	9	2

Puzzle #63 - Medium

5	4	6	3	9	7	2	8	1
7	1	2	4	8	5	3	6	9
8	9	3	6	1	2	7	5	4
4	6	7	2	5	1	9	3	8
3	5	8	7	4	9	6	1	2
1	2	9	8	6	3	4	7	5
6	7	1	9	2	8	5	4	3
2	3	5	1	7	4	8	9	6
9	8	4	5	3	6	1	2	7

Puzzle #64 - Medium

2	3	8	4	6	7	9	1	5
5	7	4	8	9	1	3	6	2
9	1	6	3	2	5	4	7	8
4	2	5	9	1	6	7	8	3
8	6	7	2	5	3	1	9	4
1	9	3	7	4	8	5	2	6
7	5	1	6	3	2	8	4	9
6	8	9	5	7	4	2	3	1
3	4	2	1	8	9	6	5	7

Puzzle #65 - Medium

9	8	6	1	3	5	2	7	4
3	1	2	4	8	7	5	9	6
7	5	4	9	2	6	3	1	8
1	2	9	7	6	4	8	3	5
4	6	3	5	1	8	9	2	7
8	7	5	3	9	2	4	6	1
2	9	8	6	5	1	7	4	3
6	3	7	8	4	9	1	5	2
5	4	1	2	7	3	6	8	9

Puzzle #66 - Medium

1	5	8	3	7	6	9	2	4
4	3	6	8	9	2	5	7	1
7	9	2	5	1	4	3	8	6
3	4	7	9	6	5	2	1	8
8	1	5	2	4	7	6	9	3
2	6	9	1	8	3	7	4	5
9	2	3	4	5	1	8	6	7
5	7	4	6	2	8	1	3	9
6	8	1	7	3	9	4	5	2

Puzzle #67 - Medium

3	1	4	6	7	2	8	5	9
9	5	6	8	3	1	2	7	4
7	8	2	4	9	5	1	3	6
1	4	3	7	6	8	5	9	2
5	6	8	2	1	9	7	4	3
2	9	7	5	4	3	6	8	1
6	7	9	1	5	4	3	2	8
8	3	5	9	2	6	4	1	7
4	2	1	3	8	7	9	6	5

Puzzle #68 - Medium

5	3	9	7	2	8	6	4	1
4	7	6	3	1	9	8	5	2
1	2	8	4	5	6	9	7	3
2	1	7	6	8	4	5	3	9
8	9	5	1	3	7	2	6	4
6	4	3	5	9	2	7	1	8
7	8	4	2	6	3	1	9	5
9	6	1	8	4	5	3	2	7
3	5	2	9	7	1	4	8	6

Puzzle #69 - Medium

5	1	6	4	2	9	7	3	8
7	4	8	3	5	1	6	2	9
3	9	2	6	7	8	4	1	5
1	2	3	8	9	4	5	6	7
9	7	4	5	6	2	1	8	3
6	8	5	7	1	3	2	9	4
4	6	9	1	8	5	3	7	2
8	5	1	2	3	7	9	4	6
2	3	7	9	4	6	8	5	1

Puzzle #70 - Medium

2	6	5	7	1	3	4	8	9
4	9	1	2	5	8	6	7	3
8	3	7	9	6	4	5	1	2
3	5	8	4	9	6	7	2	1
1	4	2	3	8	7	9	5	6
6	7	9	5	2	1	3	4	8
9	2	4	8	3	5	1	6	7
5	8	6	1	7	9	2	3	4
7	1	3	6	4	2	8	9	5

Puzzle #71 - Medium

2	6	4	1	7	8	9	5	3
1	8	5	4	3	9	2	7	6
3	9	7	5	6	2	1	8	4
7	5	6	3	9	1	4	2	8
4	1	9	2	8	6	7	3	5
8	3	2	7	4	5	6	9	1
5	2	3	6	1	7	8	4	9
9	7	1	8	5	4	3	6	2
6	4	8	9	2	3	5	1	7

Puzzle #72 - Medium

5	3	4	8	2	9	6	1	7
6	2	8	7	5	1	3	9	4
7	1	9	3	6	4	2	5	8
8	7	3	1	4	5	9	6	2
9	4	2	6	8	3	1	7	5
1	5	6	9	7	2	8	4	3
2	9	1	5	3	7	4	8	6
3	6	7	4	1	8	5	2	9
4	8	5	2	9	6	7	3	1

Puzzle #73 - Medium

7	8	3	1	5	2	6	4	9
5	2	6	8	4	9	1	3	7
1	4	9	7	6	3	5	8	2
3	7	1	9	8	5	4	2	6
6	5	8	3	2	4	7	9	1
4	9	2	6	1	7	3	5	8
9	6	7	4	3	8	2	1	5
8	3	5	2	7	1	9	6	4
2	1	4	5	9	6	8	7	3

Puzzle #74 - Medium

3	9	1	6	5	2	8	4	7
5	2	4	3	7	8	6	1	9
7	6	8	4	1	9	3	5	2
4	7	5	2	3	6	1	9	8
6	1	9	8	4	7	5	2	3
8	3	2	5	9	1	7	6	4
9	8	6	1	2	3	4	7	5
2	4	3	7	6	5	9	8	1
1	5	7	9	8	4	2	3	6

Puzzle #75 - Medium

2	3	5	1	7	9	8	6	4
8	9	1	4	6	2	3	5	7
6	7	4	5	3	8	1	9	2
4	1	3	2	8	6	9	7	5
7	8	2	9	5	3	6	4	1
5	6	9	7	1	4	2	3	8
3	5	6	8	2	7	4	1	9
1	4	8	3	9	5	7	2	6
9	2	7	6	4	1	5	8	3

Puzzle #76 - Medium

5	8	2	6	7	4	3	9	1
4	6	1	9	3	5	7	8	2
7	9	3	8	2	1	4	6	5
6	2	4	5	9	8	1	7	3
3	5	9	7	1	2	6	4	8
1	7	8	3	4	6	5	2	9
8	4	6	2	5	3	9	1	7
2	3	7	1	6	9	8	5	4
9	1	5	4	8	7	2	3	6

Puzzle #77 - Medium

1	5	8	3	2	7	9	4	6
4	6	2	5	1	9	7	3	8
3	9	7	8	4	6	2	1	5
9	4	6	7	5	8	1	2	3
8	2	1	4	9	3	6	5	7
5	7	3	1	6	2	8	9	4
6	8	4	9	3	1	5	7	2
7	3	9	2	8	5	4	6	1
2	1	5	6	7	4	3	8	9

Puzzle #78 - Medium

3	2	8	4	5	7	9	1	6
5	6	7	9	1	3	2	8	4
1	9	4	8	6	2	3	5	7
4	8	6	2	3	9	1	7	5
2	3	5	1	7	6	4	9	8
7	1	9	5	4	8	6	2	3
6	4	2	7	8	1	5	3	9
8	5	1	3	9	4	7	6	2
9	7	3	6	2	5	8	4	1

Puzzle #79 - Medium

8	2	3	4	5	7	9	1	6
7	6	5	9	1	3	2	8	4
4	9	1	8	6	2	3	5	7
9	1	7	5	4	8	6	2	3
6	8	4	2	3	9	1	7	5
5	3	2	1	7	6	4	9	8
3	7	9	6	2	5	8	4	1
1	5	8	3	9	4	7	6	2
2	4	6	7	8	1	5	3	9

Puzzle #80 - Medium

4	8	7	5	3	2	1	6	9
9	5	1	7	4	6	3	8	2
3	2	6	1	8	9	7	4	5
2	1	3	4	5	7	8	9	6
6	7	5	9	1	8	4	2	3
8	9	4	2	6	3	5	1	7
5	6	2	8	7	4	9	3	1
1	4	9	3	2	5	6	7	8
7	3	8	6	9	1	2	5	4

Puzzle #81 - Medium

2	3	6	4	8	9	1	5	7
7	9	5	1	6	2	3	8	4
8	1	4	5	3	7	9	2	6
6	2	8	7	9	3	4	1	5
4	7	9	8	5	1	6	3	2
1	5	3	2	4	6	7	9	8
3	8	7	6	1	5	2	4	9
5	6	1	9	2	4	8	7	3
9	4	2	3	7	8	5	6	1

Puzzle #82 - Medium

8	1	6	9	7	2	5	4	3
5	9	2	4	3	8	1	6	7
3	7	4	6	1	5	2	9	8
2	8	1	3	6	9	7	5	4
4	6	3	7	5	1	9	8	2
9	5	7	8	2	4	6	3	1
7	4	5	2	9	3	8	1	6
6	3	9	1	8	7	4	2	5
1	2	8	5	4	6	3	7	9

Puzzle #83 - Medium

2	7	4	6	9	3	8	5	1
1	3	8	7	4	5	2	9	6
9	5	6	2	1	8	3	7	4
7	9	3	4	5	2	6	1	8
4	1	5	8	6	7	9	3	2
6	8	2	1	3	9	5	4	7
5	4	1	3	8	6	7	2	9
3	6	7	9	2	4	1	8	5
8	2	9	5	7	1	4	6	3

Puzzle #84 - Medium

9	3	1	2	6	8	7	5	4
7	5	2	9	3	4	8	6	1
8	4	6	7	5	1	3	9	2
3	9	4	6	1	7	2	8	5
5	1	7	3	8	2	6	4	9
2	6	8	5	4	9	1	3	7
6	7	3	1	9	5	4	2	8
4	2	9	8	7	3	5	1	6
1	8	5	4	2	6	9	7	3

Puzzle #85 - Medium

9	2	7	5	6	3	4	1	8
1	4	8	7	2	9	5	6	3
5	6	3	1	8	4	9	7	2
4	9	5	3	7	8	1	2	6
2	7	1	9	5	6	3	8	4
8	3	6	2	4	1	7	5	9
3	5	9	6	1	2	8	4	7
6	1	4	8	9	7	2	3	5
7	8	2	4	3	5	6	9	1

Puzzle #86 - Medium

3	1	7	8	6	2	4	9	5
4	6	9	7	1	5	8	2	3
8	2	5	4	9	3	1	7	6
2	4	8	3	7	6	9	5	1
7	9	3	5	8	1	2	6	4
1	5	6	9	2	4	7	3	8
5	7	4	1	3	9	6	8	2
6	8	1	2	5	7	3	4	9
9	3	2	6	4	8	5	1	7

Puzzle #87 - Medium

4	7	5	3	2	1	8	9	6
9	3	8	7	6	4	1	2	5
6	2	1	8	9	5	3	4	7
7	5	6	9	1	8	2	3	4
2	1	9	4	3	6	5	7	8
3	8	4	2	5	7	6	1	9
1	9	7	6	8	2	4	5	3
8	4	2	5	7	3	9	6	1
5	6	3	1	4	9	7	8	2

Puzzle #88 - Medium

6	4	7	5	9	1	3	2	8
9	8	1	2	3	6	7	5	4
2	3	5	8	4	7	1	9	6
5	2	3	4	1	9	6	8	7
1	9	6	3	7	8	2	4	5
4	7	8	6	5	2	9	1	3
3	6	2	9	8	4	5	7	1
8	1	9	7	6	5	4	3	2
7	5	4	1	2	3	8	6	9

Puzzle #89 - Medium

9	7	3	6	4	5	1	8	2
1	2	6	3	9	8	4	5	7
8	5	4	2	1	7	9	6	3
4	9	7	8	5	3	2	1	6
5	1	2	7	6	4	8	3	9
6	3	8	9	2	1	5	7	4
7	4	1	5	3	2	6	9	8
3	6	5	4	8	9	7	2	1
2	8	9	1	7	6	3	4	5

Puzzle #90 - Medium

9	4	6	7	8	3	1	5	2
7	3	1	5	2	6	8	4	9
2	8	5	1	4	9	7	6	3
5	1	2	9	6	7	4	3	8
3	7	8	2	1	4	5	9	6
4	6	9	8	3	5	2	7	1
1	9	7	6	5	8	3	2	4
8	5	3	4	9	2	6	1	7
6	2	4	3	7	1	9	8	5

Puzzle #91 - Medium

9	2	6	8	4	5	3	1	7
1	4	8	6	3	7	2	9	5
3	5	7	9	2	1	8	6	4
2	8	9	3	5	4	1	7	6
5	7	1	2	6	8	9	4	3
6	3	4	1	7	9	5	8	2
8	6	3	4	9	2	7	5	1
4	1	5	7	8	3	6	2	9
7	9	2	5	1	6	4	3	8

Puzzle #92 - Medium

5	2	1	3	4	8	6	9	7
3	8	7	9	5	6	1	2	4
4	9	6	7	2	1	3	8	5
8	3	5	1	6	7	9	4	2
6	4	2	8	9	5	7	3	1
1	7	9	2	3	4	5	6	8
9	6	4	5	1	2	8	7	3
2	5	8	6	7	3	4	1	9
7	1	3	4	8	9	2	5	6

Puzzle #93 - Medium

5	8	1	6	9	4	2	7	3
7	3	2	5	1	8	4	9	6
4	9	6	7	2	3	8	1	5
8	1	3	2	5	6	9	4	7
9	2	4	3	7	1	6	5	8
6	5	7	4	8	9	1	3	2
2	6	9	1	3	5	7	8	4
1	4	5	8	6	7	3	2	9
3	7	8	9	4	2	5	6	1

Puzzle #94 - Medium

4	9	2	7	3	8	6	5	1
6	3	7	9	5	1	8	4	2
1	5	8	2	6	4	3	9	7
2	8	6	4	9	5	7	1	3
5	7	1	8	2	3	9	6	4
3	4	9	1	7	6	5	2	8
9	1	3	6	8	2	4	7	5
8	6	4	5	1	7	2	3	9
7	2	5	3	4	9	1	8	6

Puzzle #95 - Medium

1	3	9	8	6	4	5	7	2
2	8	7	9	5	1	4	3	6
5	6	4	2	3	7	8	9	1
6	2	5	7	8	3	1	4	9
7	9	8	1	4	5	2	6	3
4	1	3	6	9	2	7	5	8
8	5	2	3	7	6	9	1	4
3	7	1	4	2	9	6	8	5
9	4	6	5	1	8	3	2	7

Puzzle #96 - Medium

9	8	4	6	2	1	5	3	7
2	1	3	5	8	7	9	6	4
5	6	7	9	3	4	8	1	2
3	7	8	1	9	5	4	2	6
1	2	5	4	6	8	3	7	9
4	9	6	2	7	3	1	8	5
7	5	2	3	1	9	6	4	8
6	4	1	8	5	2	7	9	3
8	3	9	7	4	6	2	5	1

Puzzle #97 - Medium

3	2	7	5	1	8	4	6	9
8	1	5	6	9	4	2	3	7
9	6	4	7	2	3	8	5	1
6	9	2	1	3	5	7	4	8
4	5	1	8	6	7	3	9	2
7	8	3	9	4	2	5	1	6
5	7	6	4	8	9	1	2	3
1	3	8	2	5	6	9	7	4
2	4	9	3	7	1	6	8	5

Puzzle #98 - Medium

6	4	9	5	1	8	2	3	7
1	7	3	4	2	9	8	6	5
2	5	8	3	7	6	1	9	4
8	9	7	1	4	5	6	2	3
3	1	4	6	9	2	5	7	8
5	2	6	7	8	3	4	1	9
7	8	2	9	5	1	3	4	6
9	3	1	8	6	4	7	5	2
4	6	5	2	3	7	9	8	1

Puzzle #99 - Medium

7	6	5	3	2	1	4	8	9
3	8	1	4	7	9	2	5	6
4	9	2	5	8	6	3	7	1
5	1	4	2	9	3	8	6	7
9	2	6	8	4	7	1	3	5
8	3	7	6	1	5	9	4	2
6	4	9	1	5	8	7	2	3
2	7	3	9	6	4	5	1	8
1	5	8	7	3	2	6	9	4

Puzzle #100 - Medium

7	3	2	1	6	9	5	4	8
6	4	8	2	5	3	1	7	9
5	1	9	4	8	7	3	6	2
3	9	7	8	2	1	6	5	4
1	6	4	9	3	5	8	2	7
2	8	5	6	7	4	9	1	3
4	2	6	5	9	8	7	3	1
8	7	1	3	4	6	2	9	5
9	5	3	7	1	2	4	8	6

Puzzle #101 - Medium

2	1	5	4	6	9	7	3	8
9	8	4	3	1	7	5	6	2
3	7	6	8	5	2	1	9	4
1	2	7	6	9	4	8	5	3
8	4	3	1	2	5	9	7	6
6	5	9	7	8	3	2	4	1
5	9	8	2	4	6	3	1	7
7	6	1	5	3	8	4	2	9
4	3	2	9	7	1	6	8	5

Puzzle #102 - Medium

3	5	9	2	1	6	7	4	8
6	1	4	7	9	8	5	3	2
7	8	2	5	3	4	1	9	6
4	9	5	8	7	3	6	2	1
2	7	1	6	5	9	4	8	3
8	3	6	1	4	2	9	5	7
1	4	8	9	2	7	3	6	5
5	6	3	4	8	1	2	7	9
9	2	7	3	6	5	8	1	4

Puzzle #103 - Medium

8	9	7	3	5	2	1	4	6
6	1	2	4	7	8	5	9	3
4	3	5	9	1	6	8	2	7
1	8	4	7	2	9	6	3	5
7	2	9	6	3	5	4	8	1
5	6	3	1	8	4	2	7	9
2	4	1	5	9	7	3	6	8
3	7	8	2	6	1	9	5	4
9	5	6	8	4	3	7	1	2

Puzzle #104 - Medium

5	4	7	1	2	6	8	3	9
8	1	2	9	7	3	5	6	4
6	9	3	8	5	4	7	2	1
9	6	8	7	4	1	2	5	3
2	7	1	3	6	5	9	4	8
4	3	5	2	8	9	6	1	7
3	8	9	5	1	2	4	7	6
7	5	4	6	3	8	1	9	2
1	2	6	4	9	7	3	8	5

Puzzle #105 - Medium

8	3	9	4	7	6	5	2	1
7	5	2	1	3	9	4	6	8
6	4	1	5	8	2	9	7	3
5	6	7	3	9	4	1	8	2
9	8	4	2	6	1	3	5	7
2	1	3	8	5	7	6	9	4
3	7	8	9	1	5	2	4	6
1	2	5	6	4	8	7	3	9
4	9	6	7	2	3	8	1	5

Puzzle #106 - Medium

6	3	4	2	9	8	5	1	7
8	1	2	4	7	5	6	9	3
5	7	9	1	6	3	2	4	8
3	9	6	5	4	2	8	7	1
4	5	7	6	8	1	9	3	2
2	8	1	9	3	7	4	6	5
1	6	8	3	5	4	7	2	9
9	2	5	7	1	6	3	8	4
7	4	3	8	2	9	1	5	6

Puzzle #107 - Medium

4	2	9	1	3	7	6	5	8
3	7	6	2	8	5	9	4	1
5	1	8	6	9	4	3	7	2
9	5	1	7	2	8	4	6	3
8	6	4	9	1	3	5	2	7
2	3	7	4	5	6	8	1	9
6	9	2	3	4	1	7	8	5
1	4	5	8	7	9	2	3	6
7	8	3	5	6	2	1	9	4

Puzzle #108 - Medium

2	9	7	6	3	1	8	4	5
6	8	3	4	9	5	7	2	1
1	4	5	2	7	8	3	9	6
5	6	4	3	8	9	2	1	7
7	2	8	1	6	4	9	5	3
9	3	1	5	2	7	4	6	8
3	1	9	7	4	6	5	8	2
4	7	6	8	5	2	1	3	9
8	5	2	9	1	3	6	7	4

Puzzle #109 - Medium

5	7	4	6	2	8	1	9	3
9	3	2	5	7	1	6	8	4
6	8	1	3	9	4	2	7	5
2	4	8	9	1	5	3	6	7
7	9	3	2	4	6	5	1	8
1	5	6	7	8	3	9	4	2
3	1	7	4	5	9	8	2	6
8	2	5	1	6	7	4	3	9
4	6	9	8	3	2	7	5	1

Puzzle #110 - Medium

8	3	9	7	4	5	6	2	1
7	2	1	3	9	6	4	5	8
5	6	4	2	1	8	3	7	9
2	5	3	8	6	9	1	4	7
9	4	8	1	7	2	5	6	3
6	1	7	5	3	4	9	8	2
4	7	6	9	8	3	2	1	5
3	8	5	6	2	1	7	9	4
1	9	2	4	5	7	8	3	6

Puzzle #111 - Medium

3	5	6	4	8	1	9	7	2
7	9	2	3	6	5	4	1	8
8	1	4	9	2	7	5	6	3
6	8	3	1	4	2	7	5	9
1	2	7	6	5	9	3	8	4
5	4	9	8	7	3	1	2	6
2	7	8	5	3	4	6	9	1
9	3	5	2	1	6	8	4	7
4	6	1	7	9	8	2	3	5

Puzzle #112 - Medium

8	9	3	1	5	2	4	6	7
1	6	2	3	7	4	5	9	8
5	4	7	8	6	9	1	2	3
7	1	9	4	3	5	2	8	6
3	5	6	7	2	8	9	4	1
2	8	4	9	1	6	3	7	5
6	7	5	2	4	3	8	1	9
4	3	8	6	9	1	7	5	2
9	2	1	5	8	7	6	3	4

Puzzle #113 - Medium

3	1	4	2	8	6	5	9	7
9	6	5	7	1	4	8	2	3
2	8	7	9	5	3	1	6	4
6	5	3	8	2	7	9	4	1
7	2	9	6	4	1	3	5	8
8	4	1	3	9	5	6	7	2
4	7	6	5	3	8	2	1	9
1	9	8	4	6	2	7	3	5
5	3	2	1	7	9	4	8	6

Puzzle #114 - Medium

3	1	2	8	4	9	7	5	6
4	9	7	5	2	6	3	1	8
5	6	8	7	3	1	4	2	9
7	2	3	9	6	4	1	8	5
9	4	6	1	5	8	2	3	7
1	8	5	2	7	3	6	9	4
2	3	9	6	8	7	5	4	1
8	7	4	3	1	5	9	6	2
6	5	1	4	9	2	8	7	3

Puzzle #115 - Medium

9	3	8	5	2	1	7	4	6
5	1	6	4	7	3	9	8	2
2	7	4	6	8	9	1	5	3
6	8	2	1	5	4	3	9	7
4	9	1	2	3	7	5	6	8
3	5	7	8	9	6	2	1	4
1	6	3	7	4	5	8	2	9
7	2	5	9	6	8	4	3	1
8	4	9	3	1	2	6	7	5

Puzzle #116 - Medium

2	1	9	7	6	4	8	3	5
7	3	5	9	8	1	2	6	4
4	8	6	3	2	5	9	7	1
3	5	8	2	9	7	1	4	6
6	7	2	4	1	8	5	9	3
9	4	1	5	3	6	7	2	8
8	2	3	6	5	9	4	1	7
5	9	7	1	4	3	6	8	2
1	6	4	8	7	2	3	5	9

Puzzle #117 - Medium

5	4	1	3	2	9	8	6	7
8	7	3	5	6	1	9	4	2
9	6	2	7	8	4	1	3	5
6	9	4	8	1	5	7	2	3
2	3	7	4	9	6	5	1	8
1	8	5	2	7	3	6	9	4
7	5	6	1	3	2	4	8	9
3	1	8	9	4	7	2	5	6
4	2	9	6	5	8	3	7	1

Puzzle #118 - Medium

4	1	2	5	3	7	8	9	6
7	9	3	8	6	2	1	5	4
8	6	5	9	4	1	2	3	7
6	4	7	3	9	8	5	2	1
3	5	1	7	2	4	6	8	9
2	8	9	1	5	6	4	7	3
9	2	8	6	1	3	7	4	5
5	7	6	4	8	9	3	1	2
1	3	4	2	7	5	9	6	8

Puzzle #119 - Medium

8	9	5	3	7	4	1	6	2
7	6	4	1	5	2	8	9	3
3	2	1	8	6	9	5	4	7
4	3	6	5	8	7	9	2	1
2	5	7	6	9	1	4	3	8
9	1	8	2	4	3	6	7	5
1	4	9	7	2	8	3	5	6
6	8	2	4	3	5	7	1	9
5	7	3	9	1	6	2	8	4

Puzzle #120 - Medium

4	8	9	3	2	1	7	5	6
3	7	1	5	8	6	4	2	9
2	5	6	4	7	9	3	1	8
7	2	3	1	5	8	6	9	4
5	1	8	9	6	4	2	3	7
6	9	4	7	3	2	1	8	5
9	4	2	6	1	5	8	7	3
8	6	7	2	9	3	5	4	1
1	3	5	8	4	7	9	6	2

Puzzle #121 - Medium

7	1	9	4	6	8	3	5	2
3	5	8	2	9	1	7	4	6
6	4	2	7	5	3	9	1	8
4	6	1	3	8	5	2	7	9
9	3	5	6	2	7	4	8	1
2	8	7	9	1	4	5	6	3
8	2	6	5	7	9	1	3	4
5	9	3	1	4	6	8	2	7
1	7	4	8	3	2	6	9	5

Puzzle #122 - Medium

7	1	9	4	6	8	3	5	2
3	5	8	2	9	1	7	4	6
6	4	2	7	5	3	9	1	8
4	6	1	3	8	5	2	7	9
9	3	5	6	2	7	4	8	1
2	8	7	9	1	4	5	6	3
8	2	6	5	7	9	1	3	4
5	9	3	1	4	6	8	2	7
1	7	4	8	3	2	6	9	5

Puzzle #123 - Medium

3	1	9	7	5	4	8	2	6
4	6	8	3	9	2	1	7	5
5	2	7	8	6	1	4	9	3
9	4	3	2	8	5	7	6	1
1	7	5	6	4	9	2	3	8
6	8	2	1	3	7	9	5	4
8	5	1	9	7	3	6	4	2
2	9	4	5	1	6	3	8	7
7	3	6	4	2	8	5	1	9

Puzzle #124 - Medium

5	9	6	7	4	1	3	8	2
4	3	1	2	6	8	7	5	9
7	2	8	9	3	5	4	1	6
6	4	7	5	8	3	9	2	1
2	5	3	1	9	7	6	4	8
8	1	9	4	2	6	5	7	3
1	8	4	3	5	9	2	6	7
9	7	2	6	1	4	8	3	5
3	6	5	8	7	2	1	9	4

Puzzle #125 - Medium

1	2	9	8	5	7	6	4	3
5	7	6	4	2	3	8	9	1
8	3	4	9	6	1	7	2	5
2	6	1	7	3	4	5	8	9
3	9	8	5	1	2	4	7	6
7	4	5	6	8	9	1	3	2
6	5	3	2	7	8	9	1	4
4	8	2	1	9	6	3	5	7
9	1	7	3	4	5	2	6	8

Puzzle #126 - Medium

5	3	2	9	6	1	7	4	8
1	8	9	5	4	7	6	3	2
7	4	6	2	8	3	1	9	5
6	9	1	4	5	2	8	7	3
8	7	4	1	3	9	2	5	6
3	2	5	8	7	6	9	1	4
4	5	7	6	9	8	3	2	1
9	1	8	3	2	4	5	6	7
2	6	3	7	1	5	4	8	9

Puzzle #127 - Medium

6	3	7	5	2	1	9	8	4
2	9	8	4	3	7	1	6	5
5	4	1	8	9	6	3	2	7
1	2	9	3	5	8	4	7	6
4	6	3	2	7	9	8	5	1
8	7	5	6	1	4	2	3	9
3	1	2	9	6	5	7	4	8
9	8	6	7	4	2	5	1	3
7	5	4	1	8	3	6	9	2

Puzzle #128 - Medium

1	8	5	9	7	4	6	2	3
3	7	9	8	2	6	4	5	1
6	2	4	3	5	1	7	8	9
2	1	6	5	9	7	3	4	8
7	5	3	4	1	8	9	6	2
9	4	8	6	3	2	1	7	5
5	6	1	7	8	3	2	9	4
8	3	7	2	4	9	5	1	6
4	9	2	1	6	5	8	3	7

Puzzle #129 - Medium

9	1	3	5	4	7	6	8	2
7	8	6	9	3	2	4	1	5
2	4	5	6	1	8	7	9	3
4	9	2	1	8	5	3	6	7
6	3	8	7	2	9	5	4	1
1	5	7	4	6	3	8	2	9
5	7	4	2	9	6	1	3	8
8	2	1	3	7	4	9	5	6
3	6	9	8	5	1	2	7	4

Puzzle #130 - Medium

1	6	5	4	2	9	8	7	3
7	3	9	1	8	5	4	2	6
2	8	4	6	7	3	1	9	5
3	7	1	2	6	8	5	4	9
8	5	2	3	9	4	6	1	7
4	9	6	5	1	7	3	8	2
5	4	7	9	3	1	2	6	8
6	1	8	7	5	2	9	3	4
9	2	3	8	4	6	7	5	1

Puzzle #131 - Medium

4	8	2	9	5	1	6	7	3
5	6	1	7	3	8	4	2	9
9	3	7	2	6	4	1	8	5
7	4	5	6	8	2	9	3	1
8	1	6	3	4	9	7	5	2
3	2	9	5	1	7	8	4	6
1	7	3	4	9	5	2	6	8
6	9	4	8	2	3	5	1	7
2	5	8	1	7	6	3	9	4

Puzzle #132 - Medium

8	2	5	6	3	7	4	1	9
3	7	1	4	9	8	2	5	6
4	9	6	5	2	1	8	7	3
9	1	7	2	4	3	5	6	8
5	8	3	1	7	6	9	4	2
2	6	4	8	5	9	7	3	1
6	4	9	7	1	2	3	8	5
7	3	8	9	6	5	1	2	4
1	5	2	3	8	4	6	9	7

Puzzle #133 - Medium

3	7	9	5	4	1	6	2	8
5	8	6	3	7	2	4	1	9
2	4	1	9	6	8	3	7	5
4	1	3	6	8	9	7	5	2
8	9	2	4	5	7	1	3	6
6	5	7	1	2	3	8	9	4
1	3	5	8	9	6	2	4	7
9	2	8	7	3	4	5	6	1
7	6	4	2	1	5	9	8	3

Puzzle #134 - Medium

4	9	5	7	3	1	6	2	8
1	7	6	5	8	2	9	3	4
8	2	3	9	4	6	1	5	7
5	1	7	2	9	3	4	8	6
3	4	9	1	6	8	5	7	2
6	8	2	4	5	7	3	9	1
9	5	1	8	2	4	7	6	3
2	6	4	3	7	9	8	1	5
7	3	8	6	1	5	2	4	9

Puzzle #135 - Medium

6	4	5	9	1	8	3	7	2
3	9	1	7	2	5	6	4	8
8	7	2	3	6	4	5	1	9
5	2	8	1	4	9	7	6	3
7	1	3	8	5	6	2	9	4
4	6	9	2	7	3	1	8	5
9	8	7	6	3	2	4	5	1
1	3	4	5	8	7	9	2	6
2	5	6	4	9	1	8	3	7

Puzzle #136 - Medium

7	8	5	1	4	6	9	3	2
2	1	9	5	8	3	6	7	4
6	4	3	7	9	2	1	5	8
4	5	1	9	6	8	7	2	3
3	6	7	2	1	5	4	8	9
9	2	8	3	7	4	5	6	1
8	9	6	4	2	7	3	1	5
5	7	4	8	3	1	2	9	6
1	3	2	6	5	9	8	4	7

Puzzle #137 - Medium

2	6	9	8	5	3	1	7	4
5	4	1	6	9	7	2	8	3
8	7	3	4	1	2	6	5	9
7	2	6	3	4	1	5	9	8
3	1	8	9	6	5	7	4	2
9	5	4	7	2	8	3	6	1
4	3	5	2	7	9	8	1	6
6	8	7	1	3	4	9	2	5
1	9	2	5	8	6	4	3	7

Puzzle #138 - Medium

4	9	6	3	7	2	5	1	8
3	7	8	5	9	1	6	4	2
1	2	5	8	6	4	9	3	7
7	5	2	9	1	3	8	6	4
6	4	1	2	5	8	3	7	9
8	3	9	6	4	7	1	2	5
5	6	7	4	3	9	2	8	1
2	1	3	7	8	5	4	9	6
9	8	4	1	2	6	7	5	3

Puzzle #139 - Medium

1	6	9	5	4	3	2	8	7
5	2	3	7	8	9	4	1	6
7	8	4	2	6	1	9	5	3
3	5	6	9	7	2	8	4	1
8	4	1	3	5	6	7	2	9
2	9	7	4	1	8	3	6	5
6	1	2	8	3	7	5	9	4
9	7	5	1	2	4	6	3	8
4	3	8	6	9	5	1	7	2

Puzzle #140 - Medium

2	6	9	7	8	3	5	1	4
3	4	8	5	1	6	2	9	7
5	7	1	4	9	2	3	6	8
8	5	2	1	7	9	4	3	6
7	1	6	3	5	4	9	8	2
4	9	3	2	6	8	1	7	5
6	8	4	9	2	1	7	5	3
1	3	7	8	4	5	6	2	9
9	2	5	6	3	7	8	4	1

Puzzle 141 - Medium

3	1	6	2	9	7	8	4	5
7	8	2	1	4	5	3	9	6
9	5	4	6	8	3	7	2	1
1	3	9	8	5	2	6	7	4
4	6	7	3	1	9	5	8	2
5	2	8	4	7	6	1	3	9
2	7	5	9	3	1	4	6	8
6	4	1	7	2	8	9	5	3
8	9	3	5	6	4	2	1	7

Puzzle #142 - Medium

9	4	2	7	3	1	5	6	8
8	3	1	5	2	6	4	9	7
6	7	5	8	4	9	3	1	2
4	6	9	2	7	3	1	8	5
7	2	3	1	5	8	9	4	6
5	1	8	9	6	4	7	2	3
2	9	6	3	1	5	8	7	4
3	8	7	4	9	2	6	5	1
1	5	4	6	8	7	2	3	9

Puzzle #143 - Medium

8	3	7	9	5	6	4	2	1
9	4	6	7	2	1	5	8	3
2	5	1	3	4	8	7	9	6
3	8	5	1	6	7	2	4	9
4	6	2	8	9	5	1	3	7
7	1	9	2	3	4	8	6	5
5	2	8	6	7	3	9	1	4
1	7	3	4	8	9	6	5	2
6	9	4	5	1	2	3	7	8

Puzzle #144 - Medium

6	4	5	8	1	2	3	7	9
3	9	8	5	4	7	6	2	1
2	1	7	6	9	3	4	5	8
7	6	4	3	8	9	2	1	5
9	2	1	7	5	4	8	3	6
8	5	3	1	2	6	7	9	4
1	7	6	4	3	5	9	8	2
5	3	2	9	6	8	1	4	7
4	8	9	2	7	1	5	6	3

Puzzle #145 - Medium

6	7	1	2	5	8	9	3	4
3	2	8	6	9	4	1	5	7
5	9	4	1	7	3	6	2	8
2	8	6	7	4	5	3	9	1
7	1	5	3	2	9	4	8	6
9	4	3	8	1	6	5	7	2
4	6	2	9	3	7	8	1	5
1	5	9	4	8	2	7	6	3
8	3	7	5	6	1	2	4	9

Puzzle #146 - Medium

3	8	7	9	6	4	2	1	5
9	4	1	2	5	8	3	7	6
6	2	5	7	1	3	9	8	4
4	1	2	3	8	7	6	5	9
7	6	9	5	2	1	8	4	3
5	3	8	4	9	6	1	2	7
1	7	3	6	4	2	5	9	8
8	5	6	1	7	9	4	3	2
2	9	4	8	3	5	7	6	1

Puzzle #147 - Medium

9	7	2	8	3	4	6	1	5
1	4	5	9	2	6	3	8	7
6	8	3	1	5	7	2	9	4
7	5	1	3	4	9	8	6	2
8	2	9	6	7	1	4	5	3
3	6	4	2	8	5	9	7	1
5	3	7	4	6	8	1	2	9
4	1	8	5	9	2	7	3	6
2	9	6	7	1	3	5	4	8

Puzzle #148 - Medium

9	2	7	4	8	5	3	6	1
4	1	5	9	3	6	7	2	8
8	6	3	2	7	1	9	4	5
6	5	4	1	2	7	8	3	9
2	7	8	5	9	3	6	1	4
3	9	1	6	4	8	2	5	7
1	3	9	8	5	2	4	7	6
7	4	6	3	1	9	5	8	2
5	8	2	7	6	4	1	9	3

Puzzle #149 - Medium

7	1	3	5	8	9	4	2	6
9	2	4	7	1	6	3	5	8
5	8	6	4	2	3	7	9	1
6	7	9	8	3	4	2	1	5
3	5	8	1	7	2	9	6	4
1	4	2	6	9	5	8	7	3
4	9	1	3	6	7	5	8	2
8	3	7	2	5	1	6	4	9
2	6	5	9	4	8	1	3	7

Puzzle #150 - Medium

2	9	3	8	6	4	7	1	5
5	8	4	1	9	7	2	6	3
1	6	7	3	5	2	9	4	8
6	5	2	7	3	9	4	8	1
3	4	9	5	1	8	6	7	2
7	1	8	4	2	6	3	5	9
4	7	5	2	8	3	1	9	6
9	3	1	6	7	5	8	2	4
8	2	6	9	4	1	5	3	7

Puzzle #151 - Medium

3	7	6	1	4	9	2	5	8
2	1	5	7	8	3	9	6	4
9	8	4	5	2	6	7	1	3
6	5	9	2	1	4	3	8	7
1	2	7	8	3	5	4	9	6
8	4	3	9	6	7	5	2	1
4	3	2	6	5	8	1	7	9
5	9	8	3	7	1	6	4	2
7	6	1	4	9	2	8	3	5

Puzzle #152 - Medium

2	6	1	7	4	3	9	8	5
7	4	5	6	9	8	2	3	1
3	9	8	5	2	1	6	7	4
6	5	3	2	8	7	4	1	9
9	1	7	3	5	4	8	6	2
4	8	2	1	6	9	7	5	3
1	2	9	8	7	5	3	4	6
5	7	6	4	3	2	1	9	8
8	3	4	9	1	6	5	2	7

Puzzle #153 - Medium

8	6	5	7	3	1	9	4	2
2	1	3	8	4	9	6	7	5
7	9	4	5	2	6	8	3	1
9	3	2	6	8	7	1	5	4
4	7	8	3	1	5	2	9	6
1	5	6	4	9	2	3	8	7
5	8	1	2	7	3	4	6	9
6	4	9	1	5	8	7	2	3
3	2	7	9	6	4	5	1	8

Puzzle #154- Medium

1	6	9	4	2	5	8	7	3
4	8	7	1	9	3	2	5	6
5	3	2	8	6	7	9	1	4
3	2	6	7	5	1	4	8	9
8	9	1	3	4	2	5	6	7
7	4	5	6	8	9	3	2	1
9	1	8	5	7	4	6	3	2
6	7	4	2	3	8	1	9	5
2	5	3	9	1	6	7	4	8

Puzzle #155 - Medium

1	9	6	5	7	3	2	4	8
2	7	8	1	4	9	3	6	5
3	4	5	6	8	2	7	9	1
9	6	1	2	5	7	4	8	3
8	5	7	4	3	6	9	1	2
4	2	3	9	1	8	6	5	7
5	1	2	7	6	4	8	3	9
7	3	4	8	9	5	1	2	6
6	8	9	3	2	1	5	7	4

Puzzle 156 - Medium

8	9	2	6	7	1	3	4	5
4	1	7	2	3	5	6	9	8
6	5	3	9	8	4	7	2	1
2	6	1	8	9	3	4	5	7
5	4	8	7	1	2	9	6	3
7	3	9	5	4	6	1	8	2
9	7	4	3	5	8	2	1	6
3	8	6	1	2	9	5	7	4
1	2	5	4	6	7	8	3	9

Puzzle #157 - Medium

5	7	4	1	2	8	6	9	3
8	9	2	3	4	6	5	1	7
3	6	1	7	9	5	2	4	8
6	1	7	2	5	9	3	8	4
4	5	3	6	8	1	7	2	9
9	2	8	4	3	7	1	5	6
1	8	6	5	7	4	9	3	2
2	4	5	9	6	3	8	7	1
7	3	9	8	1	2	4	6	5

Puzzle #158 - Medium

5	4	9	3	1	6	8	2	7
2	6	7	5	8	9	1	4	3
1	8	3	7	2	4	5	6	9
4	1	5	2	3	8	7	9	6
6	9	2	1	4	7	3	5	8
7	3	8	6	9	5	2	1	4
8	7	6	9	5	2	4	3	1
3	5	4	8	6	1	9	7	2
9	2	1	4	7	3	6	8	5

Puzzle #159 - Medium

1	7	6	5	3	2	8	9	4
2	3	9	6	8	4	5	7	1
5	4	8	9	1	7	3	2	6
6	2	5	3	7	9	1	4	8
3	9	4	1	5	8	2	6	7
7	8	1	2	4	6	9	3	5
4	5	7	8	2	3	6	1	9
9	1	3	7	6	5	4	8	2
8	6	2	4	9	1	7	5	3

Puzzle #160 - Medium

8	3	1	5	2	6	4	9	7
6	7	5	8	4	9	3	1	2
9	4	2	7	3	1	5	6	8
3	8	7	4	9	2	6	5	1
2	9	6	3	1	5	8	7	4
1	5	4	6	8	7	2	3	9
5	1	8	9	6	4	7	2	3
7	2	3	1	5	8	9	4	6
4	6	9	2	7	3	1	8	5

Puzzle #161 - Medium

2	3	6	8	5	4	7	9	1
9	8	4	6	1	7	2	5	3
7	5	1	9	2	3	4	6	8
5	7	3	2	8	6	1	4	9
8	4	2	3	9	1	5	7	6
1	6	9	7	4	5	3	8	2
6	2	7	4	3	9	8	1	5
3	9	5	1	7	8	6	2	4
4	1	8	5	6	2	9	3	7

Puzzle #162 - Medium

7	5	4	9	6	8	3	1	2
3	8	9	2	5	1	7	4	6
2	1	6	4	7	3	8	5	9
1	9	2	7	8	5	4	6	3
5	6	7	3	4	2	9	8	1
8	4	3	1	9	6	2	7	5
6	3	5	8	2	7	1	9	4
9	7	1	5	3	4	6	2	8
4	2	8	6	1	9	5	3	7

Puzzle #163 - Medium

6	5	4	1	2	7	9	3	8
2	7	8	5	9	3	4	1	6
3	9	1	6	4	8	7	5	2
1	3	9	8	5	2	6	7	4
7	4	6	3	1	9	2	8	5
5	8	2	7	6	4	3	9	1
4	1	5	9	3	6	8	2	7
9	2	7	4	8	5	1	6	3
8	6	3	2	7	1	5	4	9

Puzzle #164 - Medium

5	3	8	9	4	7	2	1	6
6	4	7	1	5	2	8	3	9
2	1	9	3	6	8	5	7	4
3	2	5	4	7	1	6	9	8
7	6	1	8	2	9	3	4	5
8	9	4	6	3	5	7	2	1
9	8	3	2	1	6	4	5	7
1	7	2	5	8	4	9	6	3
4	5	6	7	9	3	1	8	2

Puzzle #165 - Medium

7	5	1	3	2	6	8	4	9
3	4	2	8	9	1	6	5	7
6	8	9	7	4	5	2	3	1
9	1	6	2	5	3	4	7	8
5	7	4	9	1	8	3	6	2
2	3	8	6	7	4	9	1	5
1	9	3	4	8	7	5	2	6
4	2	5	1	6	9	7	8	3
8	6	7	5	3	2	1	9	4

Puzzle #166 - Medium

5	6	1	4	8	3	9	7	2
4	2	9	7	1	5	6	8	3
7	3	8	6	9	2	1	4	5
8	5	4	3	7	1	2	9	6
6	7	3	2	5	9	4	1	8
9	1	2	8	4	6	5	3	7
3	4	5	1	6	7	8	2	9
1	9	7	5	2	8	3	6	4
2	8	6	9	3	4	7	5	1

Puzzle #167 - Medium

7	3	9	8	5	1	2	4	6
2	8	4	7	3	6	9	1	5
1	6	5	2	9	4	7	8	3
4	9	6	1	7	5	8	3	2
3	7	1	6	8	2	4	5	9
8	5	2	9	4	3	1	6	7
5	4	7	3	1	9	6	2	8
9	2	3	4	6	8	5	7	1
6	1	8	5	2	7	3	9	4

Puzzle #168 - Medium

6	2	8	4	5	1	3	7	9
4	7	9	6	2	3	1	8	5
1	5	3	7	8	9	6	2	4
5	6	1	8	3	7	4	9	2
3	8	7	2	9	4	5	6	1
9	4	2	5	1	6	8	3	7
2	3	6	1	7	5	9	4	8
7	9	5	3	4	8	2	1	6
8	1	4	9	6	2	7	5	3

Puzzle #169- Medium

4	8	9	3	1	7	6	5	2
5	1	2	4	6	9	3	7	8
6	7	3	8	5	2	9	1	4
8	9	5	2	4	6	1	3	7
1	6	7	5	3	8	2	4	9
2	3	4	9	7	1	8	6	5
9	5	6	7	8	3	4	2	1
3	4	8	1	2	5	7	9	6
7	2	1	6	9	4	5	8	3

Puzzle #170 - Medium

6	4	1	9	8	7	2	5	3
7	2	8	3	4	5	6	1	9
3	9	5	1	6	2	8	7	4
2	1	7	5	9	6	3	4	8
8	6	3	4	2	1	7	9	5
4	5	9	7	3	8	1	6	2
1	8	4	2	7	9	5	3	6
9	7	2	6	5	3	4	8	1
5	3	6	8	1	4	9	2	7

Puzzle 171 - Medium

2	8	7	5	3	9	1	4	6
5	6	4	1	2	8	3	7	9
1	9	3	4	7	6	2	5	8
3	7	1	8	9	5	4	6	2
9	2	5	6	4	3	8	1	7
8	4	6	2	1	7	9	3	5
4	5	8	9	6	1	7	2	3
7	1	9	3	5	2	6	8	4
6	3	2	7	8	4	5	9	1

Puzzle #172 - Medium

5	8	3	1	6	2	4	7	9
6	7	4	3	9	8	5	2	1
2	9	1	7	4	5	6	8	3
4	6	5	8	2	1	9	3	7
1	2	7	6	3	9	8	4	5
9	3	8	5	7	4	1	6	2
3	5	2	9	8	6	7	1	4
7	1	6	4	5	3	2	9	8
8	4	9	2	1	7	3	5	6

Puzzle #173 - Medium

3	9	2	8	6	4	5	1	7
7	5	4	9	1	3	6	8	2
8	6	1	7	2	5	3	4	9
2	8	5	3	4	9	1	7	6
1	3	7	2	8	6	4	9	5
6	4	9	5	7	1	8	2	3
4	2	8	6	3	7	9	5	1
5	1	6	4	9	2	7	3	8
9	7	3	1	5	8	2	6	4

Puzzle #174 - Medium

5	4	1	9	6	7	2	3	8
8	7	3	1	4	2	6	9	5
2	6	9	5	8	3	1	4	7
1	9	2	8	5	6	4	7	3
4	3	5	7	2	9	8	6	1
6	8	7	3	1	4	9	5	2
7	2	6	4	3	1	5	8	9
3	1	8	6	9	5	7	2	4
9	5	4	2	7	8	3	1	6

Puzzle #175 - Medium

9	2	5	8	1	7	6	4	3
3	7	1	4	6	2	8	9	5
8	4	6	9	3	5	2	1	7
2	8	7	1	4	6	5	3	9
5	6	4	3	7	9	1	2	8
1	9	3	2	5	8	4	7	6
6	3	2	5	9	1	7	8	4
7	1	9	6	8	4	3	5	2
4	5	8	7	2	3	9	6	1

Puzzle #176 - Medium

4	1	9	8	2	7	3	5	6
5	8	3	6	4	1	9	2	7
7	2	6	3	9	5	1	4	8
6	4	1	9	5	3	7	8	2
9	7	5	2	8	6	4	1	3
2	3	8	7	1	4	5	6	9
8	6	4	1	7	9	2	3	5
3	5	7	4	6	2	8	9	1
1	9	2	5	3	8	6	7	4

Puzzle #177 - Medium

3	7	8	9	2	4	5	1	6
5	9	1	3	7	6	4	2	8
6	2	4	5	8	1	9	7	3
9	4	5	8	6	2	1	3	7
2	8	3	7	1	5	6	4	9
7	1	6	4	9	3	2	8	5
1	5	7	6	4	8	3	9	2
8	6	2	1	3	9	7	5	4
4	3	9	2	5	7	8	6	1

Puzzle #178 - Medium

2	1	6	8	4	3	9	5	7
9	4	8	5	7	1	3	6	2
7	5	3	2	6	9	1	4	8
1	8	5	3	2	6	7	9	4
6	2	4	9	8	7	5	3	1
3	7	9	1	5	4	2	8	6
8	3	7	6	1	5	4	2	9
4	9	2	7	3	8	6	1	5
5	6	1	4	9	2	8	7	3

Puzzle #179 - Medium

7	9	3	5	4	6	1	2	8
5	8	2	1	3	9	4	7	6
4	6	1	2	7	8	5	3	9
1	7	8	9	5	2	6	4	3
3	5	9	8	6	4	2	1	7
6	2	4	3	1	7	8	9	5
8	4	6	7	9	1	3	5	2
2	3	7	4	8	5	9	6	1
9	1	5	6	2	3	7	8	4

Puzzle #180 - Medium

3	6	4	5	1	9	2	8	7
9	1	8	3	7	2	5	6	4
7	2	5	6	4	8	1	3	9
6	3	2	4	5	1	7	9	8
4	9	1	8	3	7	6	2	5
5	8	7	9	2	6	4	1	3
1	4	9	7	6	3	8	5	2
2	7	3	1	8	5	9	4	6
8	5	6	2	9	4	3	7	1

Puzzle #181 - Medium

5	8	1	6	3	7	2	4	9
3	6	4	2	8	9	7	1	5
9	2	7	4	5	1	8	6	3
1	5	8	7	2	4	9	3	6
6	9	2	3	1	8	4	5	7
4	7	3	5	9	6	1	8	2
2	3	9	1	4	5	6	7	8
7	4	5	8	6	2	3	9	1
8	1	6	9	7	3	5	2	4

Puzzle #182 - Medium

3	7	6	5	8	1	9	2	4
5	1	4	9	2	7	3	8	6
8	9	2	3	6	4	5	7	1
7	3	9	8	1	6	4	5	2
6	2	8	7	4	5	1	3	9
4	5	1	2	3	9	8	6	7
9	6	5	4	7	3	2	1	8
2	4	7	1	5	8	6	9	3
1	8	3	6	9	2	7	4	5

Puzzle #183 - Medium

8	3	9	7	6	4	5	1	2
5	7	4	9	2	1	6	3	8
2	1	6	8	5	3	4	9	7
7	2	1	4	8	9	3	6	5
6	9	8	5	3	2	7	4	1
3	4	5	1	7	6	2	8	9
9	6	3	2	1	7	8	5	4
4	5	7	3	9	8	1	2	6
1	8	2	6	4	5	9	7	3

Puzzle #184- Medium

9	1	5	2	6	4	7	3	8
7	2	3	8	5	1	9	4	6
6	4	8	7	9	3	2	1	5
2	6	1	3	7	5	8	9	4
3	9	4	1	2	8	6	5	7
8	5	7	6	4	9	1	2	3
1	3	9	4	8	6	5	7	2
5	8	2	9	3	7	4	6	1
4	7	6	5	1	2	3	8	9

Puzzle #185 - Medium

9	7	3	4	5	6	8	2	1
6	1	8	9	2	3	5	4	7
5	2	4	8	1	7	9	3	6
2	8	9	5	7	1	3	6	4
1	3	6	2	8	4	7	5	9
4	5	7	6	3	9	1	8	2
3	4	5	7	9	2	6	1	8
8	9	2	1	6	5	4	7	3
7	6	1	3	4	8	2	9	5

Puzzle 186 - Medium

3	2	8	9	1	6	7	5	4
1	9	4	3	5	7	2	6	8
5	6	7	2	8	4	3	1	9
9	7	3	8	4	1	5	2	6
8	5	1	7	6	2	4	9	3
6	4	2	5	3	9	1	8	7
7	1	9	6	2	3	8	4	5
2	3	5	4	9	8	6	7	1
4	8	6	1	7	5	9	3	2

Puzzle #187 - Medium

9	1	5	8	3	2	7	4	6
3	6	2	4	7	5	1	8	9
4	7	8	6	1	9	5	3	2
8	4	9	1	5	7	2	6	3
6	5	7	2	4	3	9	1	8
2	3	1	9	8	6	4	5	7
7	8	3	5	2	4	6	9	1
1	9	4	7	6	8	3	2	5
5	2	6	3	9	1	8	7	4

Puzzle #188 - Medium

3	9	8	5	2	1	4	6	7
7	4	5	6	9	8	1	2	3
2	6	1	7	4	3	5	9	8
6	5	3	2	8	7	9	4	1
4	8	2	1	6	9	3	7	5
9	1	7	3	5	4	2	8	6
8	3	4	9	1	6	7	5	2
1	2	9	8	7	5	6	3	4
5	7	6	4	3	2	8	1	9

Puzzle #189 - Medium

4	1	3	7	2	5	9	6	8
6	5	7	8	4	9	3	1	2
8	9	2	1	6	3	7	4	5
3	7	9	6	8	2	1	5	4
2	4	1	3	5	7	8	9	6
5	8	6	4	9	1	2	3	7
1	3	5	2	7	4	6	8	9
7	6	4	9	3	8	5	2	1
9	2	8	5	1	6	4	7	3

Puzzle #190 - Medium

3	6	7	9	5	2	8	4	1
2	9	1	6	4	8	7	5	3
4	8	5	1	7	3	6	2	9
6	2	8	4	3	9	1	7	5
5	3	4	7	6	1	9	8	2
7	1	9	8	2	5	4	3	6
8	7	3	2	9	6	5	1	4
9	4	2	5	1	7	3	6	8
1	5	6	3	8	4	2	9	7

Puzzle #191 - Medium

8	7	1	5	2	9	6	4	3
9	5	3	6	4	8	2	1	7
4	2	6	1	7	3	8	9	5
5	1	9	2	3	6	7	8	4
6	4	8	9	1	7	3	5	2
7	3	2	8	5	4	9	6	1
1	6	4	7	8	2	5	3	9
2	8	5	3	9	1	4	7	6
3	9	7	4	6	5	1	2	8

Puzzle #192 - Medium

7	8	3	5	6	9	1	2	4
6	9	4	2	1	7	3	8	5
1	2	5	4	8	3	6	9	7
8	5	2	7	3	6	4	1	9
4	6	9	1	2	5	8	7	3
3	1	7	8	9	4	2	5	6
2	4	6	9	5	8	7	3	1
9	7	1	3	4	2	5	6	8
5	3	8	6	7	1	9	4	2

Puzzle #193 - Medium

7	9	2	1	8	4	5	3	6
5	3	6	9	7	2	4	8	1
1	4	8	5	3	6	9	2	7
9	6	5	2	1	7	3	4	8
2	1	4	8	6	3	7	9	5
3	8	7	4	5	9	1	6	2
8	7	9	6	4	1	2	5	3
4	5	3	7	2	8	6	1	9
6	2	1	3	9	5	8	7	4

Puzzle #194 - Medium

1	5	2	9	8	4	6	7	3
7	4	3	1	6	5	2	8	9
6	8	9	3	2	7	5	1	4
4	6	1	2	3	9	8	5	7
8	3	5	4	7	6	1	9	2
9	2	7	8	5	1	4	3	6
2	7	4	5	1	3	9	6	8
5	9	6	7	4	8	3	2	1
3	1	8	6	9	2	7	4	5

Puzzle #195 - Medium

5	3	1	6	4	2	9	8	7
2	8	6	3	9	7	1	5	4
7	9	4	1	5	8	3	2	6
8	7	3	5	1	6	4	9	2
6	1	5	4	2	9	7	3	8
4	2	9	8	7	3	6	1	5
3	6	2	9	8	4	5	7	1
1	4	8	7	3	5	2	6	9
9	5	7	2	6	1	8	4	3

Puzzle #196 - Medium

8	3	9	2	1	6	5	7	4
7	2	1	5	8	4	6	3	9
5	6	4	7	9	3	8	2	1
2	5	3	4	7	1	9	8	6
9	4	8	6	3	5	2	1	7
6	1	7	8	2	9	4	5	3
3	8	5	9	4	7	1	6	2
1	9	2	3	6	8	7	4	5
4	7	6	1	5	2	3	9	8

Puzzle #197 - Medium

1	6	2	9	8	5	7	4	3
8	9	3	6	7	4	5	2	1
5	4	7	2	3	1	6	9	8
2	8	4	7	5	3	1	6	9
7	1	9	8	6	2	3	5	4
3	5	6	4	1	9	2	8	7
6	7	5	1	9	8	4	3	2
9	2	1	3	4	6	8	7	5
4	3	8	5	2	7	9	1	6

Puzzle #198 - Medium

1	8	7	6	4	2	5	9	3
4	9	3	8	5	1	7	2	6
5	2	6	9	7	3	8	1	4
6	7	1	2	3	5	4	8	9
9	3	2	4	8	6	1	5	7
8	4	5	7	1	9	6	3	2
3	1	9	5	6	7	2	4	8
7	5	4	3	2	8	9	6	1
2	6	8	1	9	4	3	7	5

Puzzle #199 - Medium

6	9	2	8	4	5	7	1	3
7	3	5	9	2	1	4	6	8
8	1	4	6	3	7	5	9	2
2	7	9	5	1	6	8	3	4
3	8	6	4	9	2	1	5	7
5	4	1	7	8	3	9	2	6
9	2	8	3	5	4	6	7	1
1	5	7	2	6	8	3	4	9
4	6	3	1	7	9	2	8	5

Puzzle #200 - Medium

5	8	3	2	1	6	9	4	7
6	7	4	8	3	9	1	5	2
2	9	1	5	7	4	3	6	8
4	6	5	1	8	2	7	9	3
9	3	8	4	5	7	2	1	6
1	2	7	9	6	3	5	8	4
3	5	2	6	9	8	4	7	1
8	4	9	7	2	1	6	3	5
7	1	6	3	4	5	8	2	9

Puzzle #1 - Hard

2	4	8	6	9	1	7	5	3
5	1	6	8	7	3	2	4	9
9	7	3	5	4	2	1	6	8
1	9	4	3	2	5	6	8	7
6	3	2	1	8	7	4	9	5
7	8	5	4	6	9	3	1	2
8	2	7	9	1	6	5	3	4
4	5	1	7	3	8	9	2	6
3	6	9	2	5	4	8	7	1

Puzzle #2 - Hard

2	1	9	4	7	8	3	5	6
8	3	5	9	1	6	7	2	4
4	6	7	2	5	3	8	1	9
5	8	4	1	3	7	6	9	2
6	2	3	8	9	5	4	7	1
7	9	1	6	2	4	5	3	8
3	4	2	7	8	1	9	6	5
1	5	6	3	4	9	2	8	7
9	7	8	5	6	2	1	4	3

Puzzle #3 - Hard

3	4	8	6	9	2	5	7	1
6	2	1	7	5	3	8	4	9
7	9	5	4	8	1	3	6	2
5	3	7	9	2	6	1	8	4
4	8	9	1	3	7	6	2	5
2	1	6	5	4	8	9	3	7
9	7	3	8	1	4	2	5	6
1	6	2	3	7	5	4	9	8
8	5	4	2	6	9	7	1	3

Puzzle #4- Hard

6	9	5	3	4	1	7	2	8
8	4	7	2	6	9	5	3	1
1	3	2	8	7	5	9	4	6
3	2	9	6	5	4	8	1	7
4	5	1	9	8	7	3	6	2
7	8	6	1	3	2	4	5	9
2	7	3	5	1	8	6	9	4
5	1	4	7	9	6	2	8	3
9	6	8	4	2	3	1	7	5

Puzzle #5 - Hard

9	4	1	2	8	3	5	7	6
2	6	7	9	1	5	4	8	3
5	8	3	4	7	6	9	2	1
3	5	9	6	2	7	1	4	8
7	2	8	1	9	4	3	6	5
6	1	4	5	3	8	7	9	2
1	3	2	8	4	9	6	5	7
4	7	5	3	6	2	8	1	9
8	9	6	7	5	1	2	3	4

Puzzle #6 - Hard

6	3	8	4	7	1	9	5	2
9	4	5	8	2	3	6	1	7
1	7	2	6	9	5	8	3	4
8	9	3	1	6	2	7	4	5
2	5	6	9	4	7	3	8	1
4	1	7	5	3	8	2	9	6
3	6	1	7	8	4	5	2	9
5	8	9	2	1	6	4	7	3
7	2	4	3	5	9	1	6	8

Puzzle #7- Hard

1	6	5	8	2	7	9	3	4
3	2	4	6	9	5	1	7	8
9	8	7	4	1	3	2	5	6
2	9	1	5	3	6	8	4	7
8	5	3	2	7	4	6	9	1
4	7	6	1	8	9	3	2	5
7	1	9	3	5	8	4	6	2
6	3	2	7	4	1	5	8	9
5	4	8	9	6	2	7	1	3

Puzzle #8- Hard

9	7	2	8	4	1	3	5	6
6	4	5	9	2	3	8	7	1
1	8	3	6	5	7	9	2	4
4	9	1	5	8	6	7	3	2
5	3	6	1	7	2	4	9	8
7	2	8	3	9	4	1	6	5
3	5	4	2	1	9	6	8	7
2	6	7	4	3	8	5	1	9
8	1	9	7	6	5	2	4	3

Puzzle #9- Hard

8	7	5	9	4	6	2	3	1
2	6	9	5	3	1	7	4	8
3	4	1	7	2	8	5	9	6
7	9	6	2	8	3	4	1	5
4	2	3	1	7	5	8	6	9
5	1	8	6	9	4	3	7	2
6	5	4	8	1	7	9	2	3
9	8	7	3	6	2	1	5	4
1	3	2	4	5	9	6	8	7

Puzzle #10- Hard

1	5	3	9	7	4	6	8	2
9	2	7	6	8	5	4	1	3
6	4	8	1	3	2	9	7	5
4	1	6	3	9	8	2	5	7
5	8	9	7	2	1	3	4	6
3	7	2	5	4	6	1	9	8
8	3	4	2	5	9	7	6	1
7	9	1	8	6	3	5	2	4
2	6	5	4	1	7	8	3	9

Puzzle #11- Hard

9	2	3	8	6	4	7	5	1
5	4	7	1	2	9	8	3	6
8	6	1	7	5	3	4	2	9
2	9	8	4	7	5	1	6	3
6	7	5	3	9	1	2	4	8
3	1	4	2	8	6	9	7	5
1	8	2	5	3	7	6	9	4
7	3	9	6	4	8	5	1	2
4	5	6	9	1	2	3	8	7

Puzzle #12- Hard

3	2	4	5	6	7	9	8	1
7	6	8	9	1	2	4	3	5
9	5	1	8	3	4	7	2	6
8	4	9	2	7	1	6	5	3
2	7	3	6	8	5	1	4	9
5	1	6	4	9	3	8	7	2
1	8	7	3	2	9	5	6	4
4	9	2	7	5	6	3	1	8
6	3	5	1	4	8	2	9	7

Puzzle #13- Hard

3	8	5	6	7	4	2	9	1
7	6	2	5	1	9	8	4	3
1	4	9	3	8	2	7	5	6
2	3	1	9	4	8	5	6	7
6	9	8	1	5	7	3	2	4
5	7	4	2	6	3	1	8	9
8	2	7	4	9	1	6	3	5
9	5	3	7	2	6	4	1	8
4	1	6	8	3	5	9	7	2

Puzzle #14- Hard

5	7	4	3	6	8	9	1	2
8	1	6	2	9	4	3	7	5
9	3	2	5	1	7	4	8	6
6	5	7	4	8	2	1	3	9
2	8	9	6	3	1	5	4	7
3	4	1	7	5	9	6	2	8
7	9	3	1	2	5	8	6	4
4	6	5	8	7	3	2	9	1
1	2	8	9	4	6	7	5	3

Puzzle #15- Hard

7	6	2	1	4	8	3	9	5
8	5	3	7	9	2	6	4	1
4	1	9	3	6	5	7	8	2
3	2	8	5	7	6	9	1	4
5	9	1	4	8	3	2	7	6
6	4	7	9	2	1	5	3	8
1	7	5	2	3	4	8	6	9
9	8	4	6	5	7	1	2	3
2	3	6	8	1	9	4	5	7

Puzzle #16- Hard

2	4	7	8	3	5	9	6	1
6	8	3	9	2	1	7	5	4
5	9	1	4	6	7	3	2	8
7	6	5	2	9	4	1	8	3
3	2	4	1	5	8	6	9	7
9	1	8	6	7	3	2	4	5
1	7	6	5	8	9	4	3	2
4	5	9	3	1	2	8	7	6
8	3	2	7	4	6	5	1	9

Puzzle #17- Hard

6	8	9	5	1	7	4	2	3
1	4	5	3	2	8	7	9	6
7	3	2	4	6	9	5	1	8
3	2	1	6	9	4	8	7	5
9	5	6	8	7	2	3	4	1
4	7	8	1	5	3	2	6	9
5	1	4	2	3	6	9	8	7
2	9	3	7	8	1	6	5	4
8	6	7	9	4	5	1	3	2

Puzzle #18- Hard

5	3	6	7	2	9	1	8	4
2	8	1	5	4	6	7	3	9
9	4	7	8	3	1	5	2	6
1	9	4	2	8	5	6	7	3
3	2	5	6	9	7	8	4	1
6	7	8	3	1	4	2	9	5
7	6	3	9	5	8	4	1	2
4	5	2	1	7	3	9	6	8
8	1	9	4	6	2	3	5	7

Puzzle #19- Hard

5	2	4	3	7	6	1	9	8
7	6	9	8	5	1	2	3	4
3	1	8	4	9	2	6	7	5
9	5	1	6	4	7	3	8	2
2	4	3	9	8	5	7	1	6
6	8	7	2	1	3	5	4	9
8	3	2	7	6	4	9	5	1
4	7	5	1	2	9	8	6	3
1	9	6	5	3	8	4	2	7

Puzzle #20- Hard

4	8	1	7	5	9	3	2	6
6	9	2	3	8	4	5	1	7
7	5	3	6	1	2	8	9	4
1	3	7	4	9	8	6	5	2
5	4	8	2	6	1	9	7	3
9	2	6	5	7	3	1	4	8
3	7	5	1	2	6	4	8	9
2	6	9	8	4	5	7	3	1
8	1	4	9	3	7	2	6	5

Puzzle #21- Hard

7	6	3	5	8	2	4	9	1
1	5	9	4	3	7	2	8	6
4	2	8	9	6	1	7	5	3
8	7	2	3	1	5	9	6	4
5	9	1	8	4	6	3	2	7
3	4	6	2	7	9	5	1	8
6	1	5	7	2	4	8	3	9
2	3	7	6	9	8	1	4	5
9	8	4	1	5	3	6	7	2

Puzzle #22- Hard

7	3	2	1	5	8	9	6	4
1	4	5	9	7	6	8	2	3
6	8	9	2	4	3	7	1	5
9	5	6	4	3	1	2	7	8
3	2	1	7	8	5	4	9	6
4	7	8	6	2	9	3	5	1
8	6	7	3	1	2	5	4	9
5	1	4	8	9	7	6	3	2
2	9	3	5	6	4	1	8	7

Puzzle #23- Hard

2	8	4	1	9	6	3	7	5
5	9	1	7	4	3	6	2	8
6	3	7	2	5	8	1	4	9
8	4	9	3	1	5	2	6	7
1	5	6	4	7	2	9	8	3
3	7	2	8	6	9	5	1	4
7	2	8	5	3	1	4	9	6
4	6	3	9	2	7	8	5	1
9	1	5	6	8	4	7	3	2

Puzzle #24- Hard

4	5	6	1	7	8	2	3	9
8	3	1	4	2	9	5	7	6
7	2	9	6	5	3	4	1	8
3	6	5	8	9	4	7	2	1
9	1	4	2	3	7	8	6	5
2	8	7	5	6	1	9	4	3
6	7	2	9	1	5	3	8	4
1	9	8	3	4	2	6	5	7
5	4	3	7	8	6	1	9	2

Puzzle #25- Hard

2	4	8	9	3	1	6	5	7
1	6	3	7	4	5	2	8	9
9	7	5	8	2	6	3	4	1
3	8	7	1	9	2	4	6	5
6	9	4	3	5	7	1	2	8
5	1	2	4	6	8	7	9	3
7	5	1	6	8	4	9	3	2
4	2	9	5	7	3	8	1	6
8	3	6	2	1	9	5	7	4

Puzzle #26- Hard

8	5	9	4	2	1	6	7	3
3	7	1	9	8	6	5	4	2
2	6	4	3	7	5	1	8	9
7	9	6	8	1	4	2	3	5
4	1	3	2	5	9	7	6	8
5	8	2	6	3	7	9	1	4
6	4	5	7	9	3	8	2	1
9	2	7	1	4	8	3	5	6
1	3	8	5	6	2	4	9	7

Puzzle #27- Hard

9	1	5	7	4	6	3	2	8
6	7	8	3	1	2	5	9	4
2	3	4	5	8	9	7	6	1
4	5	7	9	2	1	8	3	6
1	6	9	8	3	5	4	7	2
8	2	3	4	6	7	9	1	5
7	9	6	1	5	8	2	4	3
3	8	1	2	9	4	6	5	7
5	4	2	6	7	3	1	8	9

Puzzle #28- Hard

9	2	1	6	5	4	7	8	3
5	7	3	2	8	1	4	9	6
6	8	4	9	3	7	2	1	5
2	6	8	4	1	3	5	7	9
3	1	9	5	7	6	8	4	2
4	5	7	8	9	2	3	6	1
7	3	5	1	6	8	9	2	4
8	4	6	3	2	9	1	5	7
1	9	2	7	4	5	6	3	8

Puzzle #29- Hard

5	1	6	2	3	4	7	8	9
4	8	3	7	5	9	1	2	6
9	7	2	8	1	6	5	3	4
8	2	5	9	4	3	6	1	7
7	3	4	6	8	1	9	5	2
6	9	1	5	7	2	8	4	3
3	5	8	4	6	7	2	9	1
1	6	9	3	2	8	4	7	5
2	4	7	1	9	5	3	6	8

Puzzle #30- Hard

4	9	5	2	8	3	1	7	6
7	1	2	9	6	5	3	4	8
3	6	8	7	4	1	5	2	9
6	3	1	8	7	4	2	9	5
2	7	4	5	3	9	6	8	1
8	5	9	1	2	6	7	3	4
9	8	3	6	1	2	4	5	7
1	4	7	3	5	8	9	6	2
5	2	6	4	9	7	8	1	3

Puzzle #31- Hard

9	4	7	2	6	8	3	5	1
1	2	3	5	9	7	8	4	6
6	5	8	3	4	1	7	2	9
5	6	4	8	1	9	2	7	3
3	8	9	7	2	5	6	1	4
7	1	2	6	3	4	9	8	5
2	9	5	1	7	6	4	3	8
4	7	1	9	8	3	5	6	2
8	3	6	4	5	2	1	9	7

Puzzle #32- Hard

4	6	1	5	8	3	7	2	9
9	3	5	6	7	2	1	8	4
8	7	2	1	4	9	3	5	6
2	1	3	8	9	4	6	7	5
6	8	9	7	1	5	2	4	3
5	4	7	3	2	6	8	9	1
3	5	8	4	6	7	9	1	2
7	2	6	9	5	1	4	3	8
1	9	4	2	3	8	5	6	7

Puzzle #33- Hard

1	7	4	3	8	6	9	2	5
2	5	3	9	7	1	4	8	6
9	8	6	5	4	2	1	3	7
7	4	5	2	3	8	6	9	1
8	9	1	6	5	4	3	7	2
3	6	2	7	1	9	5	4	8
6	1	9	4	2	7	8	5	3
4	3	7	8	6	5	2	1	9
5	2	8	1	9	3	7	6	4

Puzzle #34- Hard

1	6	9	5	3	8	7	2	4
8	2	3	7	6	4	1	5	9
4	5	7	1	2	9	3	6	8
7	9	6	8	5	1	4	3	2
5	4	2	3	7	6	8	9	1
3	8	1	4	9	2	5	7	6
9	1	5	6	4	7	2	8	3
6	7	8	2	1	3	9	4	5
2	3	4	9	8	5	6	1	7

Puzzle #35- Hard

7	1	4	6	3	2	8	9	5
3	8	5	7	1	9	6	2	4
9	2	6	5	4	8	1	3	7
2	4	7	8	5	3	9	1	6
1	9	8	4	7	6	2	5	3
5	6	3	2	9	1	4	7	8
8	7	2	1	6	5	3	4	9
6	5	9	3	2	4	7	8	1
4	3	1	9	8	7	5	6	2

Puzzle #36- Hard

7	6	1	8	3	2	9	5	4
4	8	3	6	5	9	1	2	7
2	9	5	4	1	7	6	8	3
1	3	8	9	7	4	2	6	5
5	7	4	1	2	6	8	3	9
6	2	9	5	8	3	4	7	1
9	5	2	7	4	8	3	1	6
8	1	6	3	9	5	7	4	2
3	4	7	2	6	1	5	9	8

Puzzle #37- Hard

1	5	8	4	2	3	9	6	7
6	7	3	8	1	9	4	2	5
2	9	4	5	6	7	8	1	3
8	3	5	7	4	2	6	9	1
9	2	1	3	8	6	5	7	4
4	6	7	1	9	5	2	3	8
5	8	9	6	7	1	3	4	2
3	1	2	9	5	4	7	8	6
7	4	6	2	3	8	1	5	9

Puzzle #38- Hard

4	6	9	7	8	2	3	5	1
7	2	3	9	5	1	8	6	4
8	1	5	4	3	6	2	9	7
2	7	6	8	9	4	1	3	5
9	3	8	1	6	5	7	4	2
5	4	1	3	2	7	6	8	9
1	9	4	6	7	3	5	2	8
3	5	7	2	4	8	9	1	6
6	8	2	5	1	9	4	7	3

Puzzle #39- Hard

1	8	5	6	4	9	2	7	3
2	3	4	1	5	7	9	6	8
9	6	7	2	3	8	5	1	4
3	2	1	4	9	5	7	8	6
5	4	6	8	7	1	3	2	9
8	7	9	3	2	6	4	5	1
4	1	3	7	8	2	6	9	5
6	9	2	5	1	3	8	4	7
7	5	8	9	6	4	1	3	2

Puzzle #40- Hard

1	2	3	7	8	5	9	4	6
6	5	9	4	3	1	7	2	8
8	7	4	6	2	9	5	3	1
3	9	2	5	6	4	8	1	7
4	1	5	8	9	7	3	6	2
7	6	8	3	1	2	4	5	9
5	4	1	9	7	6	2	8	3
9	8	6	2	4	3	1	7	5
2	3	7	1	5	8	6	9	4

Puzzle #41- Hard

4	9	3	1	7	6	5	8	2
8	6	1	5	2	9	4	7	3
7	5	2	4	3	8	1	6	9
2	3	8	7	5	4	9	1	6
9	1	5	6	8	3	7	2	4
6	4	7	9	1	2	8	3	5
5	7	9	2	6	1	3	4	8
3	2	4	8	9	7	6	5	1
1	8	6	3	4	5	2	9	7

Puzzle #42- Hard

5	6	3	9	8	4	1	7	2
4	1	9	3	2	7	5	8	6
7	8	2	6	5	1	3	9	4
1	3	8	2	4	9	6	5	7
9	2	7	5	6	3	8	4	1
6	5	4	7	1	8	9	2	3
8	9	1	4	3	2	7	6	5
3	4	5	8	7	6	2	1	9
2	7	6	1	9	5	4	3	8

Puzzle #43- Hard

6	1	8	5	3	4	2	7	9
4	3	2	7	8	9	6	1	5
9	5	7	1	2	6	3	8	4
7	6	4	2	9	1	8	5	3
5	9	1	3	6	8	7	4	2
8	2	3	4	7	5	9	6	1
1	8	6	9	5	2	4	3	7
3	4	9	6	1	7	5	2	8
2	7	5	8	4	3	1	9	6

Puzzle #44- Hard

2	8	7	9	1	4	3	5	6
9	3	4	5	7	6	2	8	1
1	5	6	2	3	8	7	4	9
4	6	5	1	9	2	8	3	7
3	1	2	7	8	5	9	6	4
7	9	8	4	6	3	1	2	5
6	2	9	8	4	7	5	1	3
8	4	1	3	5	9	6	7	2
5	7	3	6	2	1	4	9	8

Puzzle #45- Hard

9	4	5	3	8	2	6	7	1
1	7	2	5	6	9	8	4	3
6	3	8	1	4	7	9	2	5
5	8	9	6	2	1	4	3	7
7	2	4	9	3	5	1	8	6
3	6	1	4	7	8	5	9	2
2	5	6	7	9	4	3	1	8
8	9	3	2	1	6	7	5	4
4	1	7	8	5	3	2	6	9

Puzzle #46- Hard

2	4	6	1	8	5	3	9	7
3	9	1	7	2	6	8	4	5
7	5	8	4	3	9	6	1	2
1	3	9	8	5	7	4	2	6
6	2	7	3	9	4	1	5	8
4	8	5	6	1	2	7	3	9
5	7	4	2	6	1	9	8	3
8	6	2	9	4	3	5	7	1
9	1	3	5	7	8	2	6	4

Puzzle #47- Hard

3	8	1	9	5	6	2	4	7
9	5	2	4	1	7	6	3	8
4	7	6	3	8	2	1	9	5
2	3	4	8	6	1	5	7	9
8	9	5	7	2	3	4	6	1
6	1	7	5	4	9	8	2	3
7	6	8	1	9	4	3	5	2
5	2	9	6	3	8	7	1	4
1	4	3	2	7	5	9	8	6

Puzzle #48- Hard

9	2	5	8	4	1	6	3	7
1	7	3	6	5	2	4	9	8
4	6	8	9	7	3	1	5	2
5	4	9	2	8	6	7	1	3
7	8	2	3	1	5	9	4	6
6	3	1	4	9	7	2	8	5
2	9	4	7	3	8	5	6	1
8	1	7	5	6	4	3	2	9
3	5	6	1	2	9	8	7	4

Puzzle #49- Hard

1	4	3	5	9	6	2	7	8
9	6	2	7	4	8	3	5	1
5	7	8	2	3	1	4	9	6
2	3	1	6	8	7	5	4	9
7	8	9	1	5	4	6	3	2
4	5	6	9	2	3	1	8	7
6	9	7	4	1	5	8	2	3
3	2	4	8	6	9	7	1	5
8	1	5	3	7	2	9	6	4

Puzzle #50- Hard

1	2	9	7	6	4	3	5	8
3	8	4	1	5	9	7	2	6
6	7	5	8	3	2	1	9	4
5	6	3	9	4	1	8	7	2
2	9	7	3	8	5	4	6	1
8	4	1	2	7	6	9	3	5
9	1	8	6	2	3	5	4	7
4	3	2	5	1	7	6	8	9
7	5	6	4	9	8	2	1	3

Puzzle #51- Hard

6	8	2	3	9	4	7	1	5
1	9	3	8	5	7	6	4	2
7	5	4	1	2	6	8	3	9
5	7	8	9	4	3	1	2	6
9	3	1	6	7	2	4	5	8
4	2	6	5	1	8	9	7	3
2	6	7	4	3	9	5	8	1
8	4	5	2	6	1	3	9	7
3	1	9	7	8	5	2	6	4

Puzzle #52- Hard

5	8	2	7	1	6	9	3	4
4	7	3	2	5	9	6	1	8
1	6	9	3	4	8	5	2	7
6	5	1	9	8	7	2	4	3
3	4	8	6	2	1	7	9	5
2	9	7	4	3	5	8	6	1
8	3	5	1	9	2	4	7	6
9	1	6	5	7	4	3	8	2
7	2	4	8	6	3	1	5	9

Puzzle #53- Hard

5	1	9	7	6	4	3	2	8
2	7	4	5	3	8	9	6	1
6	3	8	1	2	9	7	5	4
3	4	2	8	5	1	6	9	7
9	8	1	3	7	6	2	4	5
7	5	6	4	9	2	1	8	3
8	2	3	6	4	7	5	1	9
1	6	7	9	8	5	4	3	2
4	9	5	2	1	3	8	7	6

Puzzle #54- Hard

2	3	5	7	6	4	1	9	8
4	8	7	9	1	2	5	6	3
9	6	1	5	3	8	2	4	7
7	1	8	2	4	3	6	5	9
5	2	6	8	7	9	4	3	1
3	9	4	6	5	1	8	7	2
6	4	2	1	9	7	3	8	5
8	5	9	3	2	6	7	1	4
1	7	3	4	8	5	9	2	6

Puzzle #55- Hard

7	4	1	3	6	8	5	2	9
6	9	5	4	2	7	8	1	3
2	3	8	9	1	5	7	6	4
9	5	4	2	8	3	1	7	6
3	7	2	6	4	1	9	5	8
1	8	6	7	5	9	3	4	2
8	6	3	1	7	4	2	9	5
4	1	9	5	3	2	6	8	7
5	2	7	8	9	6	4	3	1

Puzzle #56- Hard

6	7	3	4	1	9	8	2	5
5	1	9	2	6	8	3	7	4
2	4	8	7	3	5	6	1	9
3	2	7	1	5	4	9	8	6
8	9	4	6	2	7	5	3	1
1	6	5	8	9	3	2	4	7
9	5	1	3	7	2	4	6	8
4	3	6	5	8	1	7	9	2
7	8	2	9	4	6	1	5	3

Puzzle #57- Hard

5	1	2	9	8	7	6	4	3
4	9	6	1	2	3	8	7	5
7	8	3	6	5	4	9	1	2
9	7	4	5	6	1	3	2	8
1	2	8	3	4	9	7	5	6
6	3	5	8	7	2	1	9	4
8	4	9	7	3	5	2	6	1
2	6	7	4	1	8	5	3	9
3	5	1	2	9	6	4	8	7

Puzzle #58- Hard

2	3	6	4	7	5	9	8	1
9	8	4	1	3	2	7	6	5
1	7	5	8	9	6	4	2	3
4	1	9	7	2	8	5	3	6
7	6	2	3	5	9	8	1	4
8	5	3	6	1	4	2	7	9
6	4	7	5	8	3	1	9	2
3	2	8	9	4	1	6	5	7
5	9	1	2	6	7	3	4	8

Puzzle #59- Hard

5	2	8	7	6	3	4	1	9
4	3	1	9	2	5	8	6	7
7	6	9	4	8	1	5	3	2
6	5	4	3	7	9	1	2	8
9	7	2	8	1	4	6	5	3
1	8	3	2	5	6	7	9	4
3	1	7	6	9	8	2	4	5
8	9	5	1	4	2	3	7	6
2	4	6	5	3	7	9	8	1

Puzzle #60- Hard

4	7	1	8	9	5	6	3	2
6	9	2	1	3	7	5	4	8
5	3	8	6	2	4	7	1	9
8	1	9	2	5	3	4	7	6
3	5	6	4	7	8	2	9	1
7	2	4	9	1	6	8	5	3
9	6	5	7	8	1	3	2	4
2	8	7	3	4	9	1	6	5
1	4	3	5	6	2	9	8	7

Puzzle #61 - Hard

3	1	8	6	5	2	7	4	9
7	5	4	3	9	8	2	6	1
2	6	9	7	1	4	8	3	5
5	9	2	1	6	3	4	8	7
1	8	6	4	2	7	9	5	3
4	3	7	9	8	5	6	1	2
8	4	3	2	7	1	5	9	6
6	7	1	5	4	9	3	2	8
9	2	5	8	3	6	1	7	4

Puzzle #62 - Hard

8	1	5	3	2	7	6	4	9
3	2	4	8	9	6	1	5	7
6	9	7	4	5	1	2	3	8
4	5	6	9	3	2	8	7	1
2	3	1	6	7	8	4	9	5
7	8	9	1	4	5	3	2	6
9	6	2	7	8	4	5	1	3
5	7	8	2	1	3	9	6	4
1	4	3	5	6	9	7	8	2

Puzzle #63 - Hard

2	7	9	1	8	4	5	6	3
3	8	1	5	2	6	9	7	4
4	5	6	7	3	9	2	1	8
6	4	2	3	5	7	8	9	1
7	1	3	9	6	8	4	2	5
5	9	8	4	1	2	7	3	6
1	3	4	2	9	5	6	8	7
8	2	5	6	7	3	1	4	9
9	6	7	8	4	1	3	5	2

Puzzle #64 - Hard

2	5	4	1	3	6	9	8	7
9	6	8	2	4	7	3	5	1
3	7	1	9	8	5	4	6	2
5	3	2	4	7	9	8	1	6
4	8	7	5	6	1	2	9	3
6	1	9	3	2	8	7	4	5
7	2	5	8	1	4	6	3	9
1	4	6	7	9	3	5	2	8
8	9	3	6	5	2	1	7	4

Puzzle #65 - Hard

9	7	2	3	6	5	1	8	4
6	5	4	8	1	2	7	3	9
1	8	3	4	7	9	5	2	6
7	6	9	2	5	3	8	4	1
4	3	1	7	8	6	2	9	5
5	2	8	9	4	1	6	7	3
8	9	5	6	3	7	4	1	2
3	1	7	5	2	4	9	6	8
2	4	6	1	9	8	3	5	7

Puzzle #66 - Hard

6	2	3	5	8	4	7	1	9
4	5	7	6	1	9	2	3	8
9	1	8	3	2	7	6	5	4
2	8	5	7	4	6	1	9	3
3	7	4	2	9	1	8	6	5
1	9	6	8	3	5	4	2	7
8	6	9	1	7	3	5	4	2
7	4	1	9	5	2	3	8	6
5	3	2	4	6	8	9	7	1

Puzzle #67 - Hard

8	4	6	3	5	2	1	7	9
2	9	5	4	7	1	6	8	3
3	1	7	6	8	9	2	4	5
5	8	3	9	1	6	7	2	4
1	2	9	7	3	4	5	6	8
6	7	4	8	2	5	3	9	1
9	6	1	5	4	7	8	3	2
7	3	2	1	9	8	4	5	6
4	5	8	2	6	3	9	1	7

Puzzle #68 - Hard

5	2	8	1	9	3	4	7	6
4	3	7	8	6	5	9	2	1
6	1	9	4	2	7	3	8	5
7	4	5	2	3	8	1	6	9
3	6	2	7	1	9	8	5	4
8	9	1	6	5	4	2	3	7
1	7	4	3	8	6	5	9	2
2	5	3	9	7	1	6	4	8
9	8	6	5	4	2	7	1	3

Puzzle #69 - Hard

2	8	3	7	6	4	1	5	9
9	4	5	3	2	1	7	8	6
6	1	7	5	9	8	3	4	2
7	2	4	8	5	3	6	9	1
1	5	9	4	7	6	2	3	8
3	6	8	9	1	2	5	7	4
4	3	2	1	8	5	9	6	7
8	9	1	6	3	7	4	2	5
5	7	6	2	4	9	8	1	3

Puzzle #70 - Hard

5	4	9	1	3	2	7	6	8
3	8	2	4	7	6	1	9	5
7	1	6	8	5	9	3	2	4
6	7	5	9	2	4	8	3	1
2	3	4	5	1	8	9	7	6
1	9	8	7	6	3	4	5	2
9	5	1	6	4	7	2	8	3
4	2	7	3	8	5	6	1	9
8	6	3	2	9	1	5	4	7

Puzzle #71 - Hard

1	4	8	2	6	7	5	3	9
3	6	5	9	1	4	2	7	8
7	9	2	3	5	8	1	6	4
8	1	9	6	3	2	7	4	5
2	3	4	5	7	1	9	8	6
6	5	7	4	8	9	3	1	2
9	2	1	7	4	6	8	5	3
5	7	6	8	2	3	4	9	1
4	8	3	1	9	5	6	2	7

Puzzle #72 - Hard

9	1	8	5	7	6	3	4	2
7	4	5	8	3	2	1	6	9
6	3	2	9	1	4	8	5	7
5	8	4	3	2	9	7	1	6
2	7	9	6	5	1	4	8	3
3	6	1	7	4	8	9	2	5
1	5	3	2	8	7	6	9	4
8	2	6	4	9	3	5	7	1
4	9	7	1	6	5	2	3	8

Puzzle #73 - Hard

8	3	2	9	1	5	6	4	7
1	9	6	4	7	2	3	8	5
4	7	5	8	3	6	2	9	1
9	5	1	3	2	8	4	7	6
2	4	3	7	6	1	8	5	9
6	8	7	5	9	4	1	3	2
7	6	9	2	4	3	5	1	8
3	1	8	6	5	7	9	2	4
5	2	4	1	8	9	7	6	3

Puzzle #74 - Hard

8	2	5	3	9	7	1	6	4
9	3	6	4	1	8	7	5	2
4	7	1	2	5	6	8	3	9
2	6	4	5	8	9	3	1	7
7	8	9	6	3	1	2	4	5
1	5	3	7	4	2	9	8	6
5	4	7	8	2	3	6	9	1
6	1	8	9	7	4	5	2	3
3	9	2	1	6	5	4	7	8

Puzzle #75 - Hard

4	5	9	7	3	1	6	2	8
8	7	2	9	6	4	5	3	1
3	6	1	2	5	8	7	4	9
5	3	6	8	4	7	9	1	2
1	8	7	3	9	2	4	5	6
9	2	4	5	1	6	8	7	3
2	9	5	6	7	3	1	8	4
6	4	8	1	2	5	3	9	7
7	1	3	4	8	9	2	6	5

Puzzle #76 - Hard

3	9	4	2	5	8	7	6	1
2	5	7	9	1	6	3	8	4
1	6	8	3	4	7	2	9	5
6	8	1	7	2	9	4	5	3
9	7	5	8	3	4	6	1	2
4	2	3	1	6	5	9	7	8
7	4	6	5	8	3	1	2	9
8	3	2	6	9	1	5	4	7
5	1	9	4	7	2	8	3	6

Puzzle #77 - Hard

6	7	4	8	3	5	9	2	1
3	8	2	4	1	9	5	7	6
5	1	9	6	7	2	4	8	3
9	4	8	3	2	1	6	5	7
1	5	7	9	6	8	2	3	4
2	6	3	7	5	4	8	1	9
4	9	1	2	8	7	3	6	5
8	3	5	1	4	6	7	9	2
7	2	6	5	9	3	1	4	8

Puzzle #78 - Hard

5	2	7	8	3	9	6	4	1
9	1	8	6	5	4	2	3	7
4	3	6	1	7	2	9	5	8
2	5	4	3	8	6	1	7	9
6	7	1	9	2	5	4	8	3
3	8	9	7	4	1	5	2	6
8	6	2	4	9	7	3	1	5
7	9	5	2	1	3	8	6	4
1	4	3	5	6	8	7	9	2

Puzzle #79 - Hard

3	2	4	7	1	5	6	8	9
6	9	7	8	2	3	1	4	5
8	1	5	9	6	4	7	3	2
7	8	9	6	3	2	5	1	4
2	3	1	5	4	9	8	6	7
4	5	6	1	8	7	2	9	3
9	6	2	3	5	1	4	7	8
1	4	3	2	7	8	9	5	6
5	7	8	4	9	6	3	2	1

Puzzle #80 - Hard

6	8	9	7	3	2	5	1	4
1	3	5	4	8	9	2	6	7
7	4	2	5	1	6	9	8	3
2	9	7	6	4	3	8	5	1
8	6	4	1	9	5	7	3	2
3	5	1	2	7	8	4	9	6
9	1	6	8	2	4	3	7	5
4	7	3	9	5	1	6	2	8
5	2	8	3	6	7	1	4	9

Puzzle #81 - Hard

3	4	9	6	7	2	1	5	8
6	2	1	4	5	8	7	3	9
8	7	5	1	9	3	4	2	6
2	1	6	5	4	7	9	8	3
9	3	4	8	2	6	5	7	1
5	8	7	9	3	1	2	6	4
1	5	8	2	6	4	3	9	7
7	6	2	3	1	9	8	4	5
4	9	3	7	8	5	6	1	2

Puzzle #82 - Hard

3	5	7	1	2	8	4	9	6
1	9	2	4	6	5	7	8	3
4	6	8	7	9	3	2	1	5
9	3	1	6	5	7	8	4	2
8	2	6	3	4	1	5	7	9
7	4	5	2	8	9	3	6	1
5	7	3	8	1	6	9	2	4
6	8	4	9	3	2	1	5	7
2	1	9	5	7	4	6	3	8

Puzzle #83 - Hard

8	2	4	7	5	3	6	1	9
9	5	1	2	8	6	3	7	4
3	6	7	4	9	1	8	2	5
6	4	3	5	1	8	7	9	2
1	9	5	3	2	7	4	6	8
2	7	8	9	6	4	1	5	3
4	8	9	6	7	2	5	3	1
7	3	2	1	4	5	9	8	6
5	1	6	8	3	9	2	4	7

Puzzle #84 - Hard

8	3	7	9	2	6	4	1	5
6	1	9	5	3	4	8	7	2
4	5	2	8	7	1	3	9	6
5	2	3	6	8	7	1	4	9
9	6	4	3	1	2	7	5	8
7	8	1	4	9	5	6	2	3
2	4	5	1	6	8	9	3	7
1	9	6	7	5	3	2	8	4
3	7	8	2	4	9	5	6	1

Puzzle #85 - Hard

3	2	5	8	7	6	4	1	9
9	6	8	3	1	4	5	2	7
7	4	1	9	5	2	8	6	3
1	5	9	6	4	7	2	3	8
6	8	3	2	9	5	7	4	1
2	7	4	1	3	8	6	9	5
4	1	6	5	8	9	3	7	2
5	9	7	4	2	3	1	8	6
8	3	2	7	6	1	9	5	4

Puzzle #86 - Hard

5	1	6	2	9	4	8	3	7
2	4	8	7	3	5	6	1	9
9	7	3	1	8	6	5	2	4
6	3	2	4	5	9	1	7	8
7	8	5	3	2	1	4	9	6
1	9	4	6	7	8	3	5	2
8	2	7	5	4	3	9	6	1
3	6	9	8	1	7	2	4	5
4	5	1	9	6	2	7	8	3

Puzzle #87 - Hard

2	3	4	8	6	9	7	1	5
8	1	9	4	5	7	3	2	6
6	5	7	1	2	3	8	9	4
9	2	1	5	3	8	4	6	7
5	7	6	9	1	4	2	3	8
4	8	3	2	7	6	9	5	1
7	9	2	6	4	1	5	8	3
3	6	5	7	8	2	1	4	9
1	4	8	3	9	5	6	7	2

Puzzle #88 - Hard

6	7	8	3	1	2	9	5	4
1	4	5	8	9	7	2	6	3
9	3	2	5	6	4	7	1	8
8	9	6	2	4	3	5	7	1
4	5	1	9	7	6	3	8	2
3	2	7	1	5	8	4	9	6
7	8	4	6	2	9	1	3	5
2	1	3	7	8	5	6	4	9
5	6	9	4	3	1	8	2	7

Puzzle #89 - Hard

9	2	7	5	3	8	4	1	6
6	5	3	1	9	4	8	2	7
4	8	1	6	2	7	9	5	3
1	9	8	3	6	2	5	7	4
3	4	2	7	5	1	6	9	8
5	7	6	8	4	9	2	3	1
8	3	4	9	1	5	7	6	2
2	1	9	4	7	6	3	8	5
7	6	5	2	8	3	1	4	9

Puzzle #90 - Hard

7	5	9	2	8	6	3	4	1
4	8	2	3	9	1	6	5	7
6	3	1	4	7	5	2	8	9
9	4	6	5	3	7	1	2	8
8	7	3	9	1	2	4	6	5
1	2	5	6	4	8	7	9	3
5	1	7	8	6	4	9	3	2
2	9	4	7	5	3	8	1	6
3	6	8	1	2	9	5	7	4

Puzzle #91 - Hard

2	6	9	8	5	3	4	7	1
7	5	4	2	1	6	8	3	9
3	1	8	7	9	4	2	6	5
4	3	7	6	2	1	5	9	8
5	9	2	4	7	8	3	1	6
1	8	6	9	3	5	7	4	2
6	7	1	3	8	2	9	5	4
9	2	5	1	4	7	6	8	3
8	4	3	5	6	9	1	2	7

Puzzle #92 - Hard

1	2	5	4	8	6	3	7	9
8	7	3	1	2	9	5	4	6
9	4	6	3	7	5	8	1	2
6	3	1	7	5	4	9	2	8
7	5	9	8	6	2	1	3	4
4	8	2	9	1	3	7	6	5
3	6	8	2	9	1	4	5	7
2	9	4	5	3	7	6	8	1
5	1	7	6	4	8	2	9	3

Puzzle #93 - Hard

5	6	2	3	9	8	1	4	7
1	9	7	2	4	5	6	8	3
4	3	8	6	1	7	5	2	9
6	1	4	5	7	2	9	3	8
9	8	5	4	6	3	2	7	1
2	7	3	9	8	1	4	5	6
7	2	9	1	3	4	8	6	5
3	5	1	8	2	6	7	9	4
8	4	6	7	5	9	3	1	2

Puzzle #94 - Hard

2	5	7	1	4	8	6	9	3
9	3	8	5	2	6	1	4	7
4	6	1	9	3	7	5	8	2
3	2	5	7	9	4	8	6	1
1	9	6	2	8	3	7	5	4
8	7	4	6	1	5	2	3	9
7	1	3	8	5	9	4	2	6
6	8	9	4	7	2	3	1	5
5	4	2	3	6	1	9	7	8

Puzzle #95 - Hard

4	6	3	8	5	9	7	2	1
9	8	1	7	3	2	5	4	6
5	7	2	1	4	6	3	9	8
2	4	5	9	7	1	8	6	3
3	9	8	6	2	5	4	1	7
6	1	7	3	8	4	2	5	9
7	5	9	4	6	8	1	3	2
1	3	4	2	9	7	6	8	5
8	2	6	5	1	3	9	7	4

Puzzle #96 - Hard

6	5	7	1	3	9	2	8	4
2	8	9	5	4	7	1	3	6
3	4	1	6	2	8	9	5	7
8	1	6	3	7	5	4	9	2
5	7	4	9	1	2	8	6	3
9	3	2	4	8	6	7	1	5
4	6	5	2	9	1	3	7	8
1	2	8	7	5	3	6	4	9
7	9	3	8	6	4	5	2	1

Puzzle #97 - Hard

2	7	6	8	1	4	9	3	5
8	9	4	5	3	7	1	6	2
3	1	5	6	9	2	7	8	4
9	4	7	1	6	5	8	2	3
6	5	3	2	7	8	4	9	1
1	8	2	9	4	3	6	5	7
7	3	8	4	5	6	2	1	9
4	6	9	3	2	1	5	7	8
5	2	1	7	8	9	3	4	6

Puzzle #98 - Hard

4	9	6	8	2	7	5	1	3
7	3	2	5	1	9	6	4	8
8	5	1	3	6	4	9	7	2
3	7	5	4	8	2	1	6	9
1	4	9	7	3	6	2	8	5
6	2	8	1	9	5	7	3	4
5	1	4	2	7	3	8	9	6
2	6	7	9	4	8	3	5	1
9	8	3	6	5	1	4	2	7

Puzzle #99 - Hard

7	8	5	2	1	3	4	6	9
1	9	2	5	6	4	7	3	8
4	6	3	8	9	7	5	2	1
2	3	8	6	5	1	9	4	7
9	1	4	7	8	2	6	5	3
5	7	6	4	3	9	1	8	2
8	4	7	9	2	6	3	1	5
6	2	1	3	7	5	8	9	4
3	5	9	1	4	8	2	7	6

Puzzle #100 - Hard

1	5	6	8	2	3	9	7	4
2	8	7	4	9	1	6	3	5
9	3	4	6	5	7	1	2	8
3	1	2	5	7	8	4	9	6
4	6	5	2	1	9	7	8	3
7	9	8	3	4	6	5	1	2
6	2	9	7	8	4	3	5	1
5	7	3	1	6	2	8	4	9
8	4	1	9	3	5	2	6	7

Puzzle #101 - Hard

5	9	3	7	4	2	6	8	1
1	6	2	5	9	8	7	3	4
8	4	7	3	1	6	2	9	5
3	8	5	4	7	1	9	6	2
4	7	9	2	6	5	8	1	3
6	2	1	8	3	9	4	5	7
7	1	4	6	8	3	5	2	9
9	5	6	1	2	7	3	4	8
2	3	8	9	5	4	1	7	6

Puzzle #102 - Hard

4	2	5	7	3	9	6	1	8
9	1	6	4	8	2	5	7	3
7	3	8	1	6	5	4	2	9
3	8	7	5	1	4	2	9	6
5	4	2	6	9	3	7	8	1
1	6	9	2	7	8	3	5	4
2	5	3	9	4	1	8	6	7
6	9	4	8	5	7	1	3	2
8	7	1	3	2	6	9	4	5

Puzzle #1 - Expert

4	9	1	3	7	8	6	2	5
7	8	6	5	4	2	9	3	1
3	2	5	9	1	6	8	4	7
8	5	3	1	2	4	7	9	6
9	6	4	8	5	7	3	1	2
2	1	7	6	9	3	4	5	8
1	4	8	2	6	9	5	7	3
5	3	9	7	8	1	2	6	4
6	7	2	4	3	5	1	8	9

Puzzle #2 - Expert

3	1	4	9	6	8	5	7	2
8	7	6	3	2	5	4	9	1
9	5	2	7	4	1	8	3	6
1	3	8	2	7	4	6	5	9
6	4	7	1	5	9	2	8	3
2	9	5	6	8	3	7	1	4
5	8	9	4	1	6	3	2	7
4	2	3	5	9	7	1	6	8
7	6	1	8	3	2	9	4	5

Puzzle #3 - Expert

2	8	5	1	7	6	9	3	4
9	6	1	4	3	8	5	2	7
3	7	4	5	2	9	6	1	8
5	3	8	9	1	2	4	7	6
6	1	9	7	5	4	3	8	2
4	2	7	6	8	3	1	5	9
8	4	3	2	6	1	7	9	5
1	5	6	8	9	7	2	4	3
7	9	2	3	4	5	8	6	1

Puzzle #4 - Expert

8	2	3	1	4	5	6	9	7
7	1	5	6	8	9	3	2	4
9	6	4	7	3	2	8	1	5
1	8	7	2	9	3	4	5	6
6	3	2	5	1	4	7	8	9
5	4	9	8	6	7	2	3	1
4	9	6	3	2	1	5	7	8
2	7	8	9	5	6	1	4	3
3	5	1	4	7	8	9	6	2

Puzzle #5 - Expert

5	3	2	7	6	4	9	8	1
7	8	4	9	1	2	6	3	5
1	6	9	5	3	8	4	7	2
3	7	1	4	8	5	2	6	9
9	5	8	3	2	6	1	4	7
2	4	6	1	9	7	8	5	3
8	1	7	2	4	3	5	9	6
6	2	5	8	7	9	3	1	4
4	9	3	6	5	1	7	2	8

Puzzle #6 - Expert

2	8	5	3	9	7	1	4	6
6	3	4	5	1	2	8	7	9
1	7	9	4	8	6	2	5	3
9	2	7	8	5	4	3	6	1
3	5	1	7	6	9	4	8	2
4	6	8	1	2	3	7	9	5
5	1	3	9	4	8	6	2	7
7	4	6	2	3	5	9	1	8
8	9	2	6	7	1	5	3	4

Puzzle #7 - Expert

2	7	6	3	5	1	4	9	8
3	4	5	2	8	9	7	6	1
1	8	9	6	7	4	3	2	5
5	3	2	9	1	7	8	4	6
4	6	1	5	2	8	9	3	7
7	9	8	4	6	3	1	5	2
8	2	4	1	3	5	6	7	9
9	5	7	8	4	6	2	1	3
6	1	3	7	9	2	5	8	4

Puzzle #8 - Expert

9	8	1	2	5	6	7	4	3
7	6	2	3	4	9	1	8	5
3	4	5	1	8	7	6	9	2
4	5	7	9	6	8	3	2	1
1	2	8	7	3	4	5	6	9
6	3	9	5	1	2	4	7	8
5	9	4	8	7	1	2	3	6
2	1	6	4	9	3	8	5	7
8	7	3	6	2	5	9	1	4

Puzzle #9 - Expert

6	9	8	7	3	4	2	1	5
2	3	4	9	1	5	6	8	7
5	1	7	6	2	8	4	9	3
4	7	3	8	9	2	5	6	1
9	8	2	5	6	1	3	7	4
1	6	5	3	4	7	9	2	8
3	5	9	1	8	6	7	4	2
7	4	1	2	5	9	8	3	6
8	2	6	4	7	3	1	5	9

Puzzle #10 - Expert

2	7	6	8	4	9	1	3	5
1	8	9	5	3	2	4	6	7
3	4	5	1	7	6	9	2	8
6	1	3	4	5	8	2	7	9
8	2	4	9	6	7	5	1	3
9	5	7	3	2	1	6	8	4
7	9	8	2	1	5	3	4	6
4	6	1	7	9	3	8	5	2
5	3	2	6	8	4	7	9	1

Puzzle #11 - Expert

7	4	6	1	9	8	2	3	5
5	1	3	2	6	7	9	4	8
8	9	2	3	5	4	6	7	1
4	6	8	9	7	5	1	2	3
9	2	7	6	3	1	8	5	4
3	5	1	8	4	2	7	6	9
6	3	4	7	8	9	5	1	2
1	7	9	5	2	3	4	8	6
2	8	5	4	1	6	3	9	7

Puzzle #12 - Expert

4	9	7	2	3	8	1	6	5
5	8	2	6	1	9	7	4	3
3	1	6	4	5	7	2	9	8
2	7	5	8	9	6	4	3	1
1	3	9	5	2	4	6	8	7
8	6	4	3	7	1	9	5	2
7	2	8	9	6	3	5	1	4
6	4	1	7	8	5	3	2	9
9	5	3	1	4	2	8	7	6

Puzzle #13 - Expert

8	4	2	5	3	1	7	6	9
9	5	6	8	4	7	2	3	1
3	7	1	6	9	2	8	4	5
2	9	7	4	8	3	5	1	6
6	3	8	1	5	9	4	7	2
5	1	4	2	7	6	9	8	3
4	2	9	3	1	8	6	5	7
1	6	5	7	2	4	3	9	8
7	8	3	9	6	5	1	2	4

Puzzle #14 - Expert

2	1	3	5	9	6	8	7	4
7	9	6	4	8	2	5	1	3
8	5	4	7	3	1	6	2	9
6	7	5	2	4	9	3	8	1
3	8	9	6	1	5	7	4	2
1	4	2	8	7	3	9	5	6
9	3	8	1	5	4	2	6	7
5	6	1	9	2	7	4	3	8
4	2	7	3	6	8	1	9	5

Puzzle #15 - Expert

8	3	6	4	9	5	7	1	2
2	1	9	7	3	6	5	8	4
4	7	5	8	2	1	6	9	3
5	6	4	9	1	2	3	7	8
9	2	1	3	8	7	4	5	6
3	8	7	5	6	4	1	2	9
6	4	2	1	7	9	8	3	5
1	5	3	2	4	8	9	6	7
7	9	8	6	5	3	2	4	1

Puzzle #16 - Expert

2	5	4	9	3	8	6	7	1
8	9	3	6	7	1	4	5	2
7	1	6	5	4	2	9	8	3
3	2	9	8	5	6	1	4	7
1	7	5	4	2	3	8	9	6
4	6	8	1	9	7	2	3	5
5	4	2	3	6	9	7	1	8
9	8	7	2	1	5	3	6	4
6	3	1	7	8	4	5	2	9

Puzzle #17 - Expert

7	4	5	8	1	3	6	9	2
8	6	1	2	5	9	7	4	3
9	3	2	6	4	7	8	1	5
2	9	3	1	8	4	5	6	7
6	1	7	5	3	2	9	8	4
4	5	8	9	7	6	3	2	1
5	7	9	4	2	8	1	3	6
3	8	4	7	6	1	2	5	9
1	2	6	3	9	5	4	7	8

Puzzle #18 - Expert

8	9	1	4	7	2	6	5	3
4	7	6	9	5	3	8	2	1
2	5	3	6	1	8	9	7	4
9	3	2	7	4	1	5	8	6
1	8	4	5	2	6	3	9	7
7	6	5	3	8	9	1	4	2
3	2	7	8	6	5	4	1	9
6	1	8	2	9	4	7	3	5
5	4	9	1	3	7	2	6	8

Puzzle #19 - Expert

4	3	8	2	1	7	5	6	9
9	7	5	6	3	4	2	8	1
1	2	6	9	5	8	7	3	4
5	9	3	4	6	2	1	7	8
2	6	4	7	8	1	9	5	3
7	8	1	5	9	3	4	2	6
6	4	7	3	2	9	8	1	5
3	1	2	8	4	5	6	9	7
8	5	9	1	7	6	3	4	2

Puzzle #20 - Expert

9	5	6	2	7	4	3	1	8
4	2	8	3	1	9	5	6	7
7	1	3	6	5	8	9	2	4
2	3	7	5	8	6	1	4	9
8	6	4	9	3	1	7	5	2
5	9	1	4	2	7	8	3	6
3	7	5	8	6	2	4	9	1
1	4	2	7	9	5	6	8	3
6	8	9	1	4	3	2	7	5

Puzzle #21 - Expert

5	7	4	1	3	8	6	2	9
1	8	6	5	9	2	7	3	4
2	9	3	4	7	6	8	5	1
7	6	1	3	2	5	9	4	8
8	4	5	7	6	9	3	1	2
3	2	9	8	4	1	5	7	6
4	3	8	6	1	7	2	9	5
9	5	7	2	8	4	1	6	3
6	1	2	9	5	3	4	8	7

Puzzle #22 - Expert

1	5	3	4	8	2	7	6	9
7	8	4	5	9	6	2	3	1
2	6	9	7	3	1	8	4	5
5	9	6	8	7	3	1	2	4
8	3	1	2	4	9	6	5	7
4	7	2	6	1	5	3	9	8
3	4	8	9	2	7	5	1	6
6	2	7	1	5	4	9	8	3
9	1	5	3	6	8	4	7	2

Puzzle #23 - Expert

7	8	1	9	3	5	4	2	6
5	9	3	6	2	4	1	7	8
2	6	4	8	1	7	9	5	3
4	3	8	1	7	2	5	6	9
1	2	6	5	8	9	7	3	4
9	7	5	3	4	6	2	8	1
8	5	9	7	6	1	3	4	2
3	1	2	4	5	8	6	9	7
6	4	7	2	9	3	8	1	5

Puzzle #24 - Expert

9	3	1	5	7	6	8	2	4
8	6	5	9	4	2	3	1	7
4	2	7	3	8	1	6	5	9
6	5	8	1	9	4	7	3	2
1	9	3	7	2	5	4	6	8
7	4	2	8	6	3	1	9	5
5	7	9	6	3	8	2	4	1
3	1	4	2	5	7	9	8	6
2	8	6	4	1	9	5	7	3

Puzzle #25 - Expert

3	8	2	1	4	7	9	5	6
5	9	4	2	6	8	1	7	3
1	7	6	9	5	3	2	4	8
6	4	3	5	7	2	8	9	1
7	1	5	6	8	9	4	3	2
9	2	8	4	3	1	5	6	7
2	6	1	3	9	5	7	8	4
4	5	7	8	1	6	3	2	9
8	3	9	7	2	4	6	1	5

Puzzle #26 - Expert

2	5	3	7	6	1	9	4	8
6	9	4	2	8	3	1	7	5
8	7	1	4	5	9	3	2	6
9	8	7	3	4	5	6	1	2
1	3	5	6	9	2	7	8	4
4	6	2	8	1	7	5	3	9
3	1	6	5	2	8	4	9	7
7	4	8	9	3	6	2	5	1
5	2	9	1	7	4	8	6	3

Puzzle #27 - Expert

8	2	5	9	3	7	4	6	1
7	1	9	8	4	6	5	3	2
3	6	4	1	5	2	7	9	8
6	4	8	2	1	3	9	5	7
2	9	7	5	8	4	6	1	3
5	3	1	6	7	9	8	2	4
9	8	2	7	6	1	3	4	5
4	7	6	3	2	5	1	8	9
1	5	3	4	9	8	2	7	6

Puzzle #28 - Expert

2	5	8	4	7	3	1	6	9
7	4	9	6	1	5	3	2	8
6	3	1	9	2	8	5	4	7
1	6	4	2	3	9	8	7	5
8	7	2	1	5	4	6	9	3
3	9	5	7	8	6	4	1	2
5	2	7	3	4	1	9	8	6
9	1	3	8	6	7	2	5	4
4	8	6	5	9	2	7	3	1

Puzzle #29 - Expert

1	4	7	3	8	6	5	9	2
9	6	8	5	4	2	7	1	3
2	3	5	9	7	1	6	4	8
6	9	1	4	2	7	3	8	5
5	8	2	1	9	3	4	7	6
4	7	3	8	6	5	9	2	1
7	5	4	2	3	8	1	6	9
3	2	6	7	1	9	8	5	4
8	1	9	6	5	4	2	3	7

Puzzle #30 - Expert

2	5	7	1	3	9	4	6	8
9	4	1	6	8	5	7	3	2
6	3	8	7	2	4	1	9	5
4	2	9	8	5	6	3	1	7
8	1	3	4	7	2	6	5	9
7	6	5	9	1	3	8	2	4
1	9	4	2	6	8	5	7	3
3	8	6	5	9	7	2	4	1
5	7	2	3	4	1	9	8	6

Puzzle #31 - Expert

4	2	8	1	5	3	7	6	9
7	5	9	8	6	4	1	2	3
3	1	6	7	2	9	8	5	4
5	4	3	2	9	8	6	7	1
9	8	1	6	4	7	2	3	5
6	7	2	3	1	5	9	4	8
8	9	7	4	3	6	5	1	2
1	6	4	5	8	2	3	9	7
2	3	5	9	7	1	4	8	6

Puzzle #32 - Expert

9	1	4	8	6	3	7	2	5
6	8	3	7	2	5	9	4	1
5	2	7	1	4	9	6	3	8
8	5	6	3	1	4	2	9	7
3	7	2	9	8	6	1	5	4
4	9	1	5	7	2	3	8	6
2	6	9	4	5	7	8	1	3
7	4	8	2	3	1	5	6	9
1	3	5	6	9	8	4	7	2

Puzzle #33 - Expert

7	5	2	1	9	8	4	6	3
8	6	9	2	3	4	1	7	5
3	4	1	7	6	5	2	9	8
5	9	3	8	4	2	7	1	6
4	1	7	6	5	9	8	3	2
6	2	8	3	7	1	9	5	4
1	8	6	9	2	3	5	4	7
9	3	5	4	8	7	6	2	1
2	7	4	5	1	6	3	8	9

Puzzle #34 - Expert

5	1	9	8	6	3	2	7	4
8	4	6	7	2	5	3	1	9
2	7	3	1	9	4	8	6	5
6	9	8	2	5	7	4	3	1
1	2	4	6	3	8	9	5	7
3	5	7	4	1	9	6	2	8
4	8	2	5	7	6	1	9	3
7	3	1	9	4	2	5	8	6
9	6	5	3	8	1	7	4	2

Puzzle #35 - Expert

7	1	8	2	6	4	3	5	9
5	3	9	7	8	1	2	4	6
2	4	6	5	3	9	1	7	8
9	5	7	8	1	2	4	6	3
1	6	2	3	4	7	8	9	5
4	8	3	6	9	5	7	2	1
8	9	5	4	2	3	6	1	7
3	2	1	9	7	6	5	8	4
6	7	4	1	5	8	9	3	2

Puzzle #36 - Expert

6	8	5	7	4	1	9	3	2
2	4	1	3	8	9	7	6	5
7	9	3	5	2	6	1	8	4
5	3	7	2	9	4	6	1	8
8	6	2	1	3	7	5	4	9
9	1	4	8	6	5	3	2	7
4	7	9	6	1	8	2	5	3
3	5	6	4	7	2	8	9	1
1	2	8	9	5	3	4	7	6

Puzzle #37 - Expert

6	3	4	1	9	5	7	8	2
8	9	7	6	2	4	5	3	1
1	2	5	7	3	8	9	4	6
3	5	2	4	7	1	6	9	8
7	8	6	9	5	3	1	2	4
4	1	9	8	6	2	3	5	7
9	7	3	2	4	6	8	1	5
2	6	8	5	1	9	4	7	3
5	4	1	3	8	7	2	6	9

Puzzle #38 - Expert

9	6	8	5	2	7	1	3	4
2	4	5	9	1	3	7	8	6
7	1	3	4	8	6	2	5	9
1	9	6	2	5	8	3	4	7
3	8	2	7	4	9	5	6	1
5	7	4	6	3	1	8	9	2
8	5	7	1	6	4	9	2	3
4	2	1	3	9	5	6	7	8
6	3	9	8	7	2	4	1	5

Puzzle #39 - Expert

2	7	5	4	9	1	8	6	3
3	6	8	7	5	2	1	4	9
4	9	1	3	6	8	7	2	5
8	3	6	1	4	9	5	7	2
9	2	7	6	8	5	3	1	4
5	1	4	2	3	7	9	8	6
1	8	3	9	2	6	4	5	7
6	5	9	8	7	4	2	3	1
7	4	2	5	1	3	6	9	8

Puzzle #40 - Expert

3	2	8	5	6	9	7	4	1
5	4	9	7	3	1	8	6	2
1	6	7	4	8	2	3	5	9
6	3	4	9	1	8	2	7	5
7	5	1	3	2	4	9	8	6
9	8	2	6	7	5	1	3	4
4	7	5	2	9	3	6	1	8
8	9	3	1	5	6	4	2	7
2	1	6	8	4	7	5	9	3

Puzzle #41 - Expert

4	3	1	5	2	7	6	9	8
9	5	2	4	8	6	1	7	3
6	8	7	9	1	3	4	2	5
5	1	4	8	7	2	3	6	9
3	2	9	1	6	4	5	8	7
8	7	6	3	9	5	2	4	1
7	4	3	2	5	8	9	1	6
2	9	8	6	3	1	7	5	4
1	6	5	7	4	9	8	3	2

Puzzle #42 - Expert

9	2	3	6	7	5	8	1	4
1	6	7	8	4	9	3	5	2
5	4	8	2	1	3	7	9	6
7	5	9	3	6	1	2	4	8
8	3	4	5	9	2	6	7	1
2	1	6	7	8	4	9	3	5
4	7	5	9	2	6	1	8	3
6	8	1	4	3	7	5	2	9
3	9	2	1	5	8	4	6	7

Puzzle #43 - Expert

9	3	7	2	1	4	8	6	5
6	1	2	7	5	8	4	9	3
5	8	4	6	9	3	7	2	1
2	5	9	8	7	1	3	4	6
4	7	8	3	2	6	1	5	9
1	6	3	9	4	5	2	8	7
7	4	1	5	6	2	9	3	8
3	9	5	4	8	7	6	1	2
8	2	6	1	3	9	5	7	4

Puzzle #44 - Expert

3	9	2	5	1	8	6	7	4
8	5	4	7	9	6	3	2	1
1	6	7	2	4	3	8	9	5
6	4	3	1	8	2	9	5	7
9	8	5	4	3	7	1	6	2
2	7	1	9	6	5	4	8	3
7	1	8	3	5	9	2	4	6
4	2	6	8	7	1	5	3	9
5	3	9	6	2	4	7	1	8

Puzzle #45 - Expert

2	7	4	3	8	9	6	5	1
9	3	5	6	2	1	7	4	8
1	8	6	5	4	7	3	9	2
6	2	8	9	5	4	1	3	7
5	9	3	7	1	6	2	8	4
4	1	7	8	3	2	9	6	5
3	4	1	2	9	8	5	7	6
8	6	9	1	7	5	4	2	3
7	5	2	4	6	3	8	1	9

Puzzle #46 - Expert

8	3	2	7	4	5	1	6	9
9	4	7	8	1	6	3	5	2
1	5	6	2	9	3	8	4	7
2	6	5	1	7	4	9	8	3
4	8	1	6	3	9	2	7	5
3	7	9	5	2	8	4	1	6
6	1	3	9	8	7	5	2	4
5	9	8	4	6	2	7	3	1
7	2	4	3	5	1	6	9	8

Puzzle #47 - Expert

8	2	4	6	3	5	9	1	7
9	5	7	1	2	4	3	8	6
1	3	6	8	7	9	2	4	5
7	1	5	9	6	3	4	2	8
2	8	3	4	5	7	1	6	9
4	6	9	2	8	1	7	5	3
6	9	8	7	4	2	5	3	1
5	7	2	3	1	6	8	9	4
3	4	1	5	9	8	6	7	2

Puzzle #48 - Expert

9	3	5	1	2	4	8	6	7
7	8	2	9	3	6	5	4	1
6	1	4	7	5	8	3	9	2
2	5	7	8	6	9	4	1	3
1	9	3	5	4	2	6	7	8
8	4	6	3	1	7	9	2	5
4	7	9	2	8	3	1	5	6
3	6	1	4	7	5	2	8	9
5	2	8	6	9	1	7	3	4

Puzzle #49 - Expert

7	3	4	2	9	8	1	5	6
2	8	9	6	5	1	4	3	7
1	5	6	7	3	4	9	2	8
3	4	7	5	1	9	8	6	2
9	2	5	3	8	6	7	1	4
6	1	8	4	7	2	3	9	5
8	6	2	9	4	3	5	7	1
5	9	1	8	6	7	2	4	3
4	7	3	1	2	5	6	8	9

Puzzle #50 - Expert

2	7	1	9	6	4	3	8	5
9	6	4	3	8	5	7	2	1
5	8	3	2	7	1	4	9	6
3	5	8	7	1	9	6	4	2
1	4	6	5	2	3	9	7	8
7	2	9	8	4	6	1	5	3
4	9	5	1	3	8	2	6	7
8	1	2	6	9	7	5	3	4
6	3	7	4	5	2	8	1	9

Puzzle #51 - Expert

8	7	1	3	6	2	5	9	4
4	9	3	5	7	8	2	1	6
6	2	5	1	4	9	8	7	3
5	1	2	7	8	4	6	3	9
9	6	8	2	1	3	4	5	7
7	3	4	6	9	5	1	2	8
2	5	6	4	3	7	9	8	1
3	4	9	8	5	1	7	6	2
1	8	7	9	2	6	3	4	5

Puzzle #52 - Expert

1	8	4	9	5	6	7	2	3
9	5	2	3	4	7	8	1	6
7	6	3	8	2	1	4	5	9
5	7	6	1	3	2	9	4	8
3	4	9	7	8	5	2	6	1
2	1	8	6	9	4	5	3	7
4	3	1	2	7	8	6	9	5
8	9	5	4	6	3	1	7	2
6	2	7	5	1	9	3	8	4

Puzzle #53 - Expert

7	5	4	2	9	6	8	3	1
8	9	6	1	5	3	4	2	7
1	3	2	7	8	4	5	9	6
4	1	3	8	6	5	2	7	9
2	7	5	4	1	9	3	6	8
6	8	9	3	2	7	1	4	5
3	6	8	9	4	1	7	5	2
9	4	1	5	7	2	6	8	3
5	2	7	6	3	8	9	1	4

Puzzle #54 - Expert

9	2	5	6	8	1	7	4	3
7	3	6	9	4	5	1	2	8
1	4	8	3	7	2	6	5	9
8	5	9	2	1	7	3	6	4
6	7	2	4	3	8	9	1	5
4	1	3	5	6	9	8	7	2
5	6	7	8	9	4	2	3	1
3	9	4	1	2	6	5	8	7
2	8	1	7	5	3	4	9	6

Puzzle #1 - Extreme

4	6	1	5	7	8	9	2	3
2	8	7	3	4	9	5	1	6
3	9	5	2	1	6	7	4	8
8	1	4	6	9	5	2	3	7
9	7	3	1	2	4	6	8	5
6	5	2	7	8	3	1	9	4
5	4	9	8	6	2	3	7	1
7	2	6	4	3	1	8	5	9
1	3	8	9	5	7	4	6	2

Puzzle #2 - Extreme

7	8	3	4	6	9	5	2	1
6	5	1	2	8	7	9	4	3
4	2	9	5	1	3	6	8	7
1	3	6	7	5	4	2	9	8
8	4	7	9	2	6	1	3	5
5	9	2	8	3	1	7	6	4
2	7	5	3	9	8	4	1	6
3	6	4	1	7	2	8	5	9
9	1	8	6	4	5	3	7	2

Puzzle #3 - Extreme

9	3	4	8	6	2	7	5	1
5	1	6	7	4	3	9	8	2
7	8	2	9	1	5	3	6	4
3	6	1	5	7	4	2	9	8
8	5	9	1	2	6	4	3	7
2	4	7	3	9	8	5	1	6
6	7	3	2	5	1	8	4	9
1	2	5	4	8	9	6	7	3
4	9	8	6	3	7	1	2	5

Puzzle #4 - Extreme

7	6	3	4	2	1	9	5	8
8	2	1	9	5	3	7	4	6
4	9	5	7	6	8	3	1	2
6	5	7	2	1	9	8	3	4
2	1	8	3	7	4	5	6	9
9	3	4	5	8	6	2	7	1
1	4	2	8	3	5	6	9	7
3	7	6	1	9	2	4	8	5
5	8	9	6	4	7	1	2	3

Puzzle #5 - Extreme

3	5	4	9	6	8	7	1	2
9	7	1	3	4	2	5	6	8
6	8	2	5	7	1	4	3	9
4	3	6	7	5	9	2	8	1
8	1	5	4	2	3	9	7	6
2	9	7	1	8	6	3	5	4
1	4	9	6	3	7	8	2	5
7	6	8	2	9	5	1	4	3
5	2	3	8	1	4	6	9	7

Puzzle #6 - Extreme

6	1	3	4	7	5	2	8	9
2	5	9	1	8	3	7	4	6
7	8	4	6	9	2	1	5	3
3	7	8	9	4	6	5	1	2
9	4	2	3	5	1	6	7	8
1	6	5	7	2	8	9	3	4
5	2	7	8	3	9	4	6	1
8	9	1	5	6	4	3	2	7
4	3	6	2	1	7	8	9	5

Puzzle #7 - Extreme

1	3	5	6	8	4	7	2	9
7	8	4	2	9	5	6	3	1
6	2	9	7	3	1	4	8	5
4	1	2	8	7	9	3	5	6
5	9	3	4	2	6	8	1	7
8	7	6	1	5	3	2	9	4
9	5	8	3	6	7	1	4	2
2	6	1	5	4	8	9	7	3
3	4	7	9	1	2	5	6	8

Puzzle #8 - Extreme

1	6	5	4	9	3	2	8	7
2	3	9	7	8	5	4	6	1
4	8	7	1	6	2	3	9	5
8	5	6	2	4	1	9	7	3
3	7	2	9	5	6	8	1	4
9	4	1	8	3	7	6	5	2
5	9	8	3	1	4	7	2	6
6	2	4	5	7	9	1	3	8
7	1	3	6	2	8	5	4	9

Puzzle #9 - Extreme

5	3	1	7	8	4	9	2	6
4	6	7	2	5	9	8	3	1
8	9	2	6	1	3	7	5	4
3	4	9	1	6	5	2	8	7
1	2	5	3	7	8	4	6	9
7	8	6	9	4	2	5	1	3
9	5	8	4	3	6	1	7	2
2	7	3	8	9	1	6	4	5
6	1	4	5	2	7	3	9	8

Puzzle #10 - Extreme

2	8	7	6	5	1	9	3	4
4	6	1	3	9	2	8	5	7
3	9	5	8	7	4	6	2	1
5	4	9	1	3	7	2	8	6
1	3	8	2	4	6	7	9	5
7	2	6	9	8	5	1	4	3
6	5	2	4	1	9	3	7	8
8	1	4	7	2	3	5	6	9
9	7	3	5	6	8	4	1	2

Puzzle #11 - Extreme

6	2	9	8	5	3	7	4	1
4	8	7	9	6	1	3	5	2
3	1	5	7	2	4	6	9	8
9	4	8	3	1	7	2	6	5
1	6	2	5	4	9	8	7	3
7	5	3	6	8	2	9	1	4
2	7	1	4	3	6	5	8	9
5	3	6	1	9	8	4	2	7
8	9	4	2	7	5	1	3	6

Puzzle #12 - Extreme

3	6	2	5	1	4	8	7	9
7	1	4	8	6	9	3	2	5
9	5	8	3	7	2	1	4	6
1	4	7	9	8	5	2	6	3
8	9	5	6	2	3	7	1	4
6	2	3	7	4	1	5	9	8
2	3	9	1	5	6	4	8	7
5	7	1	4	9	8	6	3	2
4	8	6	2	3	7	9	5	1

Puzzle #13 - Extreme

4	1	9	7	5	3	6	2	8
3	7	6	9	8	2	4	1	5
8	2	5	6	4	1	7	3	9
1	8	7	3	9	4	5	6	2
9	6	4	5	2	7	3	8	1
2	5	3	8	1	6	9	7	4
6	9	2	1	3	5	8	4	7
5	3	1	4	7	8	2	9	6
7	4	8	2	6	9	1	5	3

Puzzle #14 - Extreme

8	7	4	1	6	9	5	3	2
1	5	3	4	2	7	9	6	8
2	9	6	3	5	8	4	7	1
5	3	7	2	8	6	1	9	4
6	2	1	9	4	5	7	8	3
4	8	9	7	1	3	6	2	5
7	1	2	6	3	4	8	5	9
9	4	8	5	7	2	3	1	6
3	6	5	8	9	1	2	4	7

Puzzle #15 - Extreme

6	5	1	9	4	3	8	7	2
7	8	3	5	2	1	6	9	4
4	2	9	6	8	7	1	3	5
1	3	6	2	9	8	5	4	7
5	9	2	7	6	4	3	1	8
8	4	7	1	3	5	2	6	9
2	7	5	4	1	6	9	8	3
3	6	4	8	5	9	7	2	1
9	1	8	3	7	2	4	5	6

Puzzle #16 - Extreme

7	6	9	4	1	2	8	3	5
1	3	5	8	6	7	9	2	4
4	2	8	9	5	3	6	7	1
8	4	3	2	7	1	5	6	9
9	1	6	3	8	5	2	4	7
5	7	2	6	4	9	3	1	8
2	9	4	7	3	8	1	5	6
3	5	7	1	9	6	4	8	2
6	8	1	5	2	4	7	9	3

Puzzle #17 - Extreme

1	6	3	7	2	8	4	9	5
2	5	9	6	3	4	7	8	1
4	7	8	9	1	5	2	3	6
5	8	4	1	7	2	9	6	3
9	3	7	5	8	6	1	2	4
6	1	2	3	4	9	5	7	8
8	2	6	4	5	7	3	1	9
3	9	5	2	6	1	8	4	7
7	4	1	8	9	3	6	5	2

Puzzle #18 - Extreme

4	9	5	3	2	8	7	6	1
1	8	2	6	7	9	3	5	4
7	6	3	1	4	5	8	2	9
2	1	8	9	3	7	6	4	5
6	3	4	8	5	2	1	9	7
9	5	7	4	6	1	2	8	3
8	7	9	2	1	4	5	3	6
5	2	6	7	9	3	4	1	8
3	4	1	5	8	6	9	7	2

Puzzle #19 - Extreme

8	3	4	7	6	5	1	2	9
6	9	2	3	4	1	5	8	7
7	5	1	8	2	9	4	3	6
3	1	8	2	7	6	9	4	5
2	6	5	9	3	4	8	7	1
4	7	9	1	5	8	3	6	2
1	8	6	4	9	2	7	5	3
5	4	3	6	1	7	2	9	8
9	2	7	5	8	3	6	1	4

Puzzle #20 - Extreme

2	8	5	3	4	9	1	7	6
4	7	6	1	8	5	9	2	3
9	3	1	6	7	2	8	5	4
3	9	7	4	6	1	5	8	2
1	6	8	5	2	3	4	9	7
5	4	2	7	9	8	6	3	1
8	2	4	9	3	6	7	1	5
7	1	3	8	5	4	2	6	9
6	5	9	2	1	7	3	4	8

Puzzle #21 - Extreme

9	7	1	8	5	3	2	6	4
5	4	6	9	2	7	8	1	3
8	2	3	4	1	6	7	5	9
2	9	7	3	8	5	1	4	6
6	8	4	7	9	1	5	3	2
1	3	5	6	4	2	9	7	8
3	1	9	2	7	4	6	8	5
4	5	2	1	6	8	3	9	7
7	6	8	5	3	9	4	2	1

Puzzle #22 - Extreme

8	5	9	6	1	4	7	3	2
4	1	7	5	3	2	6	8	9
2	6	3	9	8	7	1	5	4
5	9	8	4	7	1	2	6	3
7	4	1	3	2	6	8	9	5
3	2	6	8	5	9	4	7	1
9	3	2	7	4	8	5	1	6
1	7	5	2	6	3	9	4	8
6	8	4	1	9	5	3	2	7

Puzzle #23 - Extreme

5	1	9	7	6	4	3	8	2
3	8	2	9	5	1	6	4	7
6	7	4	3	8	2	1	5	9
2	3	6	1	7	8	4	9	5
4	5	8	2	3	9	7	6	1
1	9	7	6	4	5	8	2	3
8	4	1	5	9	3	2	7	6
9	6	3	8	2	7	5	1	4
7	2	5	4	1	6	9	3	8

Puzzle #24 - Extreme

1	9	6	5	3	2	7	8	4
3	8	5	4	7	1	9	2	6
4	7	2	9	6	8	5	1	3
8	1	9	2	4	7	6	3	5
6	4	3	8	5	9	1	7	2
5	2	7	3	1	6	4	9	8
2	6	8	1	9	4	3	5	7
7	3	1	6	2	5	8	4	9
9	5	4	7	8	3	2	6	1

Puzzle #25 - Extreme

2	8	5	3	6	7	1	4	9
9	6	7	1	8	4	5	2	3
4	1	3	9	2	5	7	6	8
8	2	1	5	7	9	4	3	6
5	3	4	8	1	6	2	9	7
7	9	6	2	4	3	8	1	5
6	5	8	4	3	2	9	7	1
3	4	9	7	5	1	6	8	2
1	7	2	6	9	8	3	5	4

Puzzle #26 - Extreme

8	9	6	1	4	7	2	5	3
5	4	1	6	2	3	7	9	8
3	2	7	5	8	9	4	6	1
1	6	5	3	9	2	8	7	4
4	8	9	7	1	5	3	2	6
2	7	3	8	6	4	5	1	9
7	1	4	2	3	6	9	8	5
9	5	8	4	7	1	6	3	2
6	3	2	9	5	8	1	4	7

Puzzle #27 - Extreme

8	5	9	1	2	4	6	3	7
7	4	3	5	8	6	1	9	2
1	6	2	9	3	7	4	5	8
9	2	6	4	5	8	3	7	1
4	8	7	6	1	3	9	2	5
5	3	1	7	9	2	8	6	4
6	7	8	2	4	9	5	1	3
3	9	5	8	7	1	2	4	6
2	1	4	3	6	5	7	8	9

Puzzle #28 - Extreme

2	8	9	5	4	3	7	1	6
6	4	1	9	2	7	3	8	5
7	3	5	1	8	6	2	9	4
3	2	6	4	7	9	8	5	1
8	1	7	2	6	5	4	3	9
9	5	4	3	1	8	6	7	2
1	9	2	8	3	4	5	6	7
4	6	3	7	5	1	9	2	8
5	7	8	6	9	2	1	4	3

Puzzle #29 - Extreme

6	5	9	1	2	3	8	7	4
1	7	3	5	8	4	6	2	9
2	4	8	9	7	6	5	1	3
5	6	1	8	3	9	7	4	2
9	2	4	7	6	5	3	8	1
3	8	7	4	1	2	9	5	6
4	1	5	3	9	8	2	6	7
8	3	6	2	4	7	1	9	5
7	9	2	6	5	1	4	3	8

Puzzle #30 - Extreme

1	2	5	7	3	8	4	6	9
7	8	6	4	9	2	5	1	3
3	4	9	6	1	5	2	8	7
5	3	1	8	7	4	9	2	6
4	6	7	5	2	9	8	3	1
8	9	2	1	6	3	7	5	4
2	7	3	9	8	1	6	4	5
9	5	8	3	4	6	1	7	2
6	1	4	2	5	7	3	9	8

Puzzle #31 - Extreme

2	1	4	5	8	6	7	9	3
7	5	8	3	4	9	2	6	1
6	9	3	1	7	2	4	5	8
5	6	2	8	9	3	1	7	4
1	3	9	4	5	7	6	8	2
4	8	7	2	6	1	5	3	9
9	4	5	7	2	8	3	1	6
3	2	6	9	1	5	8	4	7
8	7	1	6	3	4	9	2	5

Puzzle #32 - Extreme

6	4	9	2	5	1	3	8	7
8	2	7	4	9	3	1	5	6
1	5	3	8	6	7	9	2	4
3	8	1	6	7	4	2	9	5
2	9	6	3	1	5	7	4	8
5	7	4	9	2	8	6	3	1
4	6	5	7	3	2	8	1	9
9	3	8	1	4	6	5	7	2
7	1	2	5	8	9	4	6	3

Puzzle #33 - Extreme

8	1	6	9	4	7	3	5	2
5	2	7	3	1	8	4	6	9
3	9	4	5	2	6	7	8	1
9	8	2	4	5	1	6	7	3
7	5	3	6	8	2	9	1	4
6	4	1	7	9	3	5	2	8
2	6	9	1	3	5	8	4	7
1	3	5	8	7	4	2	9	6
4	7	8	2	6	9	1	3	5

Puzzle #34 - Extreme

8	5	4	2	1	6	3	9	7
2	9	1	3	7	4	8	5	6
7	3	6	9	8	5	2	1	4
6	4	2	5	3	9	7	8	1
3	1	5	8	6	7	4	2	9
9	8	7	4	2	1	6	3	5
4	6	8	1	5	3	9	7	2
1	7	3	6	9	2	5	4	8
5	2	9	7	4	8	1	6	3

Puzzle #35 - Extreme

5	7	4	9	8	2	3	1	6
2	9	6	3	5	1	4	8	7
3	8	1	6	4	7	9	5	2
9	3	8	1	6	4	7	2	5
4	6	5	7	2	3	1	9	8
7	1	2	5	9	8	6	3	4
1	5	3	8	7	6	2	4	9
8	2	7	4	3	9	5	6	1
6	4	9	2	1	5	8	7	3

Puzzle #36 - Extreme

5	3	8	9	6	7	4	1	2
4	2	9	5	3	1	8	6	7
1	7	6	8	2	4	9	5	3
2	8	4	7	5	3	1	9	6
3	9	7	1	8	6	5	2	4
6	5	1	4	9	2	7	3	8
7	4	2	6	1	9	3	8	5
8	1	3	2	7	5	6	4	9
9	6	5	3	4	8	2	7	1

Puzzle #37 - Extreme

7	8	9	4	1	5	2	6	3
4	1	6	2	7	3	8	5	9
2	3	5	9	6	8	4	1	7
6	2	3	5	8	9	7	4	1
9	5	8	1	4	7	3	2	6
1	7	4	3	2	6	5	9	8
3	6	2	8	9	4	1	7	5
8	4	7	6	5	1	9	3	2
5	9	1	7	3	2	6	8	4

Puzzle #38 - Extreme

5	1	4	2	7	6	8	9	3
6	3	8	1	5	9	7	4	2
2	9	7	4	8	3	1	5	6
8	4	2	5	3	1	6	7	9
3	7	1	6	9	2	4	8	5
9	5	6	8	4	7	3	2	1
1	6	5	7	2	4	9	3	8
4	2	9	3	1	8	5	6	7
7	8	3	9	6	5	2	1	4

Puzzle #39 - Extreme

2	1	8	3	6	4	5	7	9
3	4	5	9	7	2	8	1	6
9	6	7	1	5	8	2	4	3
1	3	4	6	8	7	9	2	5
6	7	9	2	3	5	1	8	4
8	5	2	4	9	1	3	6	7
5	8	6	7	1	9	4	3	2
7	2	1	5	4	3	6	9	8
4	9	3	8	2	6	7	5	1

Puzzle #40 - Extreme

5	2	8	9	1	7	6	4	3
6	1	4	8	2	3	9	7	5
3	7	9	4	6	5	2	8	1
7	9	6	5	3	4	1	2	8
2	8	3	6	7	1	4	5	9
4	5	1	2	8	9	7	3	6
1	4	2	3	5	6	8	9	7
8	6	5	7	9	2	3	1	4
9	3	7	1	4	8	5	6	2

Puzzle #41 - Extreme

5	9	6	2	7	3	4	1	8
3	8	7	1	4	9	2	5	6
4	2	1	6	5	8	3	7	9
9	4	3	5	6	1	7	8	2
8	7	5	9	3	2	1	6	4
6	1	2	7	8	4	5	9	3
7	5	9	4	2	6	8	3	1
1	3	4	8	9	5	6	2	7
2	6	8	3	1	7	9	4	5

Puzzle #42 - Extreme

2	9	7	4	1	6	8	5	3
4	5	3	8	9	2	1	6	7
8	1	6	3	5	7	9	4	2
3	8	4	9	2	1	6	7	5
5	7	1	6	3	4	2	8	9
9	6	2	7	8	5	4	3	1
1	3	8	5	4	9	7	2	6
7	4	9	2	6	3	5	1	8
6	2	5	1	7	8	3	9	4

Puzzle #43 - Extreme

4	2	6	1	3	5	8	9	7
9	1	7	6	8	4	2	5	3
8	5	3	2	9	7	6	1	4
5	3	8	9	7	1	4	2	6
2	7	9	5	4	6	3	8	1
1	6	4	8	2	3	9	7	5
7	4	2	3	1	9	5	6	8
3	9	5	7	6	8	1	4	2
6	8	1	4	5	2	7	3	9

Puzzle #44 - Extreme

1	9	5	8	7	6	2	3	4
8	2	4	3	5	9	6	1	7
6	7	3	4	1	2	5	8	9
4	5	6	7	8	3	9	2	1
2	3	7	5	9	1	4	6	8
9	8	1	6	2	4	3	7	5
7	6	2	1	4	5	8	9	3
5	1	9	2	3	8	7	4	6
3	4	8	9	6	7	1	5	2

Puzzle #45 - Extreme

7	3	9	1	2	8	6	4	5
2	5	8	3	6	4	1	9	7
1	6	4	5	9	7	2	8	3
6	8	5	4	3	1	9	7	2
3	9	7	2	5	6	4	1	8
4	1	2	7	8	9	5	3	6
9	7	6	8	1	2	3	5	4
8	2	3	9	4	5	7	6	1
5	4	1	6	7	3	8	2	9

Puzzle #46 - Extreme

6	1	2	4	5	8	3	7	9
4	7	3	1	9	2	8	6	5
5	8	9	6	3	7	2	4	1
8	4	7	9	2	5	1	3	6
3	5	1	8	6	4	9	2	7
2	9	6	3	7	1	5	8	4
9	3	5	2	4	6	7	1	8
1	2	4	7	8	9	6	5	3
7	6	8	5	1	3	4	9	2

Puzzle #47 - Extreme

7	6	1	2	9	3	5	8	4
4	9	5	1	8	7	3	6	2
8	2	3	6	5	4	9	7	1
3	8	2	7	4	6	1	9	5
1	5	9	3	2	8	7	4	6
6	4	7	9	1	5	8	2	3
5	1	4	8	7	2	6	3	9
2	7	6	5	3	9	4	1	8
9	3	8	4	6	1	2	5	7

Puzzle #48 - Extreme

4	8	1	7	3	9	6	5	2
5	6	3	2	4	1	9	8	7
9	2	7	5	6	8	1	3	4
6	5	4	9	7	3	8	2	1
2	3	8	4	1	6	7	9	5
1	7	9	8	2	5	4	6	3
7	1	6	3	8	2	5	4	9
3	4	5	6	9	7	2	1	8
8	9	2	1	5	4	3	7	6

Puzzle #49 - Extreme

7	6	3	8	4	9	1	2	5
1	2	5	3	6	7	8	4	9
9	4	8	5	1	2	6	7	3
2	8	6	4	9	3	7	5	1
5	9	1	2	7	8	3	6	4
3	7	4	6	5	1	9	8	2
8	3	9	7	2	4	5	1	6
6	1	2	9	8	5	4	3	7
4	5	7	1	3	6	2	9	8

Puzzle #50 - Extreme

2	1	7	5	9	8	6	4	3
8	3	9	1	6	4	7	5	2
5	6	4	7	2	3	1	8	9
3	5	1	8	7	6	2	9	4
7	2	8	4	3	9	5	1	6
9	4	6	2	1	5	8	3	7
4	7	5	9	8	2	3	6	1
6	9	2	3	5	1	4	7	8
1	8	3	6	4	7	9	2	5

Puzzle #51 - Extreme

2	7	6	4	1	3	8	9	5
4	5	9	8	2	6	3	1	7
3	1	8	9	7	5	4	2	6
5	6	2	7	3	8	1	4	9
7	9	3	1	4	2	6	5	8
1	8	4	6	5	9	2	7	3
6	4	1	5	8	7	9	3	2
9	3	5	2	6	1	7	8	4
8	2	7	3	9	4	5	6	1

Puzzle #52 - Extreme

5	7	8	1	3	9	6	4	2
3	9	6	8	4	2	7	1	5
4	1	2	5	6	7	8	9	3
6	4	7	2	5	8	9	3	1
9	3	5	4	7	1	2	6	8
8	2	1	3	9	6	5	7	4
2	8	9	6	1	4	3	5	7
7	5	4	9	2	3	1	8	6
1	6	3	7	8	5	4	2	9

Puzzle #53 - Extreme

9	5	8	4	3	7	2	1	6
7	4	2	5	1	6	9	3	8
1	6	3	2	9	8	7	5	4
4	3	9	7	5	1	6	8	2
2	8	7	3	6	4	1	9	5
6	1	5	9	8	2	4	7	3
5	2	1	6	7	3	8	4	9
3	7	6	8	4	9	5	2	1
8	9	4	1	2	5	3	6	7

Puzzle #54 - Extreme

4	5	9	1	6	3	2	7	8
2	6	3	4	7	8	1	9	5
7	1	8	2	5	9	3	6	4
6	2	5	7	4	1	9	8	3
8	7	4	3	9	5	6	2	1
3	9	1	8	2	6	5	4	7
9	3	6	5	8	4	7	1	2
1	4	2	9	3	7	8	5	6
5	8	7	6	1	2	4	3	9